SOMATIC EXERCISES FOR BEGINNERS

Harmonize your body and mind with simple somatic exercises for a vibrant new you

TERESA MILLER

COPYRIGHT ©
All rights reserved.

TABLE OF CONTENTS

Posture, breathing cue and awareness when practicing seated spinal twist --- 91

Step-by-step guide to Body Scan Meditation ----------- 94

Posture, breathing cue and awareness when practicing body scan meditation --- 97

INTRODUCTION

Welcome to the doorway of self-discovery and holistic wellness – the world of somatic exercises. In an era dominated by hectic schedules and constant distractions, the art of reconnecting with our bodies often gets sidelined. However, within the realm of somatic exercises lies an empowering opportunity to rediscover our innate capacity for physical ease, emotional balance, and profound self-awareness.

Somatic exercises go beyond the conventional notions of exercise; they encompass a holistic approach to wellness, delving into the interconnectedness of mind, body, and spirit. At its essence, somatic practice revolves around the idea of embodiment – a conscious journey into the depths of our physical sensations, movements, and inner experiences.

Imagine a practice that doesn't focus solely on external appearances or rigid workout structures but rather emphasizes internal exploration and self-awareness. Somatic exercises are this unique journey; they're about reacquainting yourself with your body's language, understanding its whispers and needs, and nurturing a sense of unity within yourself.

At its core, somatic practice is an embodiment of mindfulness and kinesthetic awareness. It's a gentle, introspective voyage that encourages you to listen to your body's cues, to untangle knots of tension, and to reclaim agency over your physical and emotional state.

This guide is your gateway into the world of somatic exercises – a comprehensive roadmap designed especially for beginners. Whether you're a newcomer to the concept or someone seeking a deeper connection with their physical self, this guide is poised to serve as your compass on this transformative expedition.

The potential benefits of somatic exercises are multifaceted and transformative. Develop a heightened awareness of your body's signals, allowing you to detect and address areas of tension or discomfort. Discover how somatic exercises can enhance your posture, mobility, and overall ease of movement by re-educating the body to move with efficiency and grace.

Experience the profound relaxation that comes with releasing chronic muscle tension, leading to reduced stress levels and an increased sense of calmness. Cultivate a deeper connection between your mind and body, fostering a sense of unity and balance that transcends physical movements. Harness the body's natural ability to heal itself by identifying and addressing physical imbalances or limitations.

This comprehensive guide is your gateway into the world of somatic exercises, designed to introduce beginners to this transformative practice. Here's what you can expect: Explore the core principles and philosophy behind somatic exercises, laying the groundwork for your practice. Delve into a curated selection of introductory exercises, accompanied by detailed instructions and illustrations, making the practice accessible and understandable. Progress through the guide to explore advanced exercises and variations, empowering you to deepen your somatic experience.

Learn to navigate common challenges or misconceptions, equipped with troubleshooting tips and corrective measures. Discover firsthand the array of benefits that await you on this transformative journey toward holistic well-being.

Prepare yourself for a transformative odyssey that leads you back to the sanctuary within i.e your body. By embarking on this journey of somatic exercises, you're poised to unlock a world of self-discovery, healing, and revitalization. Let this guide be your companion, guiding you toward a deeper understanding of your body and a heightened sense of well-being.

Are you ready to embark on this empowering journey? Let's commence the exploration together.

CHAPTER ONE

WHAT ARE SOMATIC EXERCISES?

Somatic exercises refer to a category of movement-based practices focused on increasing awareness of the body, improving movement patterns, releasing muscular tension, and enhancing overall physical well-being through mindful and intentional movement. The term "somatic" derives from the Greek word "soma," which means the living body as perceived from within.

Here are the key aspects that define somatic exercises:

• Mindful Movement: Somatic exercises emphasize mindful movement and awareness of bodily sensations. Practitioners learn to move with conscious attention to internal sensations rather than merely focusing on external actions.

• Re-Education of Movement Patterns: They involve re-educating the body's habitual movement patterns by releasing chronic muscular contractions or tensions. This re-education aims to restore natural and efficient movement.

• Mind-Body Connection: Somatic exercises promote a deep mind-body connection. They emphasize the understanding that physical tension or stress can be interconnected with emotional and psychological states.

• Gentle and Slow Movements: These exercises often involve slow, gentle movements, allowing individuals to explore and understand their body's responses and limitations without force or strain.

• Increased Body Awareness: They foster increased body awareness, enabling practitioners to recognize and address areas of tension, discomfort, or imbalances within their bodies.

• Various Practices: Somatic exercises encompass a range of practices and techniques, including but not limited to the Feldenkrais Method, Alexander Technique, Hanna Somatics, Body-Mind Centering, and Somatic Experiencing.

Overall, somatic exercises offer a holistic approach to wellness by facilitating a deeper understanding of the body-mind connection and empowering individuals to improve their movement patterns and overall quality of life through conscious and mindful movement practices.

THE BENEFITS OF SOMATIC EXERCISES

Somatic exercises offer a wide array of benefits that encompass physical, mental, and emotional well-being. Here are the key advantages associated with practicing somatic exercises:

1. Improved Body Awareness:

Somatic exercises cultivate a heightened sense of body awareness. Practitioners become more attuned to internal sensations, enabling them to recognize and address areas of tension, discomfort, or imbalances within their bodies.

2. Enhanced Movement Patterns:

By focusing on re-educating movement patterns, somatic exercises help individuals release chronic muscular contractions or tensions. This can lead to improved movement efficiency, coordination, and overall ease of motion.

3. Reduced Stress and Tension:

These exercises emphasize the release of chronic muscular contractions and stress-related tension, leading to reduced stress levels, increased relaxation, and an overall sense of calmness.

4. Improved Posture and Flexibility:

Through the practice of somatic exercises, individuals can experience enhanced posture, increased flexibility, and a greater range of motion. By releasing tension and encouraging optimal movement, somatic exercises contribute to better body alignment and functional movement.

5. Alleviation of Muscular Pain:

Somatic exercises can help alleviate muscular pain and discomfort by addressing underlying movement patterns and releasing tension. This may be particularly beneficial for individuals dealing with chronic pain conditions or muscle stiffness.

6. Mind-Body Integration:

Somatic practices emphasize the connection between the mind and body. By fostering a harmonious integration, practitioners can experience a greater sense of holistic well-being, mental clarity, and emotional balance.

7. Stress Reduction and Relaxation:

The mindful and gentle nature of somatic exercises promotes relaxation responses in the body, allowing individuals to unwind, reduce stress, and find moments of deep relaxation.

8. Increased Emotional Resilience:

Regular practice of somatic exercises may lead to increased emotional resilience. By addressing physical tension and promoting relaxation, practitioners often experience a more centered and balanced emotional state.

9. Rehabilitation and Injury Prevention:

Somatic exercises can aid in rehabilitation post-injury by encouraging gentle movement and re-educating the body's movement patterns. Additionally, they may help prevent injuries by promoting better body mechanics and movement awareness.

10. Overall Well-being and Quality of Life:

By integrating mindful movement into daily life, somatic exercises contribute to an overall sense of well-being, improved quality of life, and a deeper connection to one's body and self.

These benefits collectively make somatic exercises a valuable practice for anyone seeking to enhance their physical comfort, movement efficiency, stress management, and overall wellness by fostering a deeper connection between the body and mind.

SIGNIFICANCE OF SOMATIC EXERCISES

Somatic exercises hold significant importance in promoting holistic well-being and fostering a deeper understanding of the mind-body connection. Here are the key significances of somatic exercises:

1. Mind-Body Connection:

Somatic exercises emphasize the intricate relationship between the mind and body. By encouraging mindfulness and internal awareness, they facilitate a deeper understanding of how thoughts, emotions, and physical sensations interrelate.

2. Increased Body Awareness:

Practicing somatic exercises cultivates heightened body awareness. Individuals learn to perceive and respond to their body's signals, allowing them to identify areas of tension, release muscular tightness, and address imbalances.

3. Movement Re-Education:

These exercises focus on re-educating movement patterns. By releasing habitual muscular contractions and improving movement efficiency, somatic exercises can enhance posture, coordination, and overall ease of movement.

4. Stress Reduction and Relaxation:

Somatic exercises emphasize relaxation and stress reduction. By promoting gentle, mindful movements and releasing muscular tension, practitioners can activate the body's relaxation response, leading to reduced stress levels and increased relaxation.

5. Pain Management:

They offer a holistic approach to managing muscular pain and discomfort. By addressing underlying movement patterns and releasing tension, somatic exercises can be beneficial for alleviating chronic pain conditions or stiffness.

6. Improved Functionality and Flexibility:

Regular practice of somatic exercises can enhance functionality and flexibility. By optimizing movement patterns and encouraging a fuller range of motion, individuals can experience improved mobility and functional movement.

7. Rehabilitation and Injury Prevention:

Somatic exercises can aid in rehabilitation post-injury by promoting gentle movements and re-educating the body's movements. They also contribute to injury prevention by enhancing body awareness and promoting better body mechanics.

8. Emotional and Psychological Well-being:

Through the mind-body connection, somatic exercises can positively impact emotional and psychological well-being. By reducing stress, enhancing relaxation, and fostering a sense of centeredness, individuals often experience improved mental clarity and emotional balance.

9. Holistic Wellness:

These exercises contribute to holistic wellness by addressing not only physical aspects but also emotional, mental, and even spiritual dimensions. They support an integrated approach to well-being by promoting harmony between various aspects of an individual's life.

10. Empowerment and Self-Care:

Engaging in somatic exercises empowers individuals to take an active role in their health and self-care. By fostering self-awareness and providing tools for managing stress and tension, practitioners gain a sense of control and agency over their well-being.

Overall, the significance of somatic exercises lies in their ability to foster a profound mind-body connection, promote relaxation, improve movement patterns, and support overall physical, mental, and emotional wellness.

THE FUNDAMENTAL PRINCIPLES BEHIND SOMATIC EXERCISES

The fundamental principles behind somatic exercises are rooted in fostering a deeper mind-body connection, enhancing body awareness, and promoting conscious movement. These principles form the foundation of somatic practices and guide practitioners in their approach to self-discovery and holistic well-being. Here are the key principles:

1. Mindfulness and Awareness:

• Embodied Awareness: Somatic exercises emphasize being fully present in the body, cultivating a deep awareness of internal sensations, movements, and bodily responses.

• Conscious Attention: Practitioners are encouraged to pay focused attention to their bodily sensations, thoughts, emotions, and movements without judgment or distraction.

2. Sensory Perception:

• Internal Sensation: Somatic exercises prioritize exploring and understanding internal bodily sensations, such as muscle tension, breathing patterns, and subtle movements.

• Proprioception and Interoception: Developing proprioceptive (awareness of body position) and interoceptive (awareness of internal body states) abilities is integral to somatic practices.

3. Gentle and Mindful Movement:

• Slow, Deliberate Movements: Somatic exercises involve slow, intentional movements that encourage practitioners to explore sensations, promoting a deeper connection with the body.

• Non-Forceful Approach: The focus is on gentle, non-invasive movements that avoid force or strain, allowing individuals to listen to their body's cues and avoid overexertion.

4. Release of Tension and Habitual Patterns:

• Tension Release: Somatic exercises aim to release chronic muscular tension and stress patterns held within the body, enabling practitioners to let go of habitual muscular contractions.

• Re-education of Movement Patterns: By re-educating the body's movement patterns, somatic practices aim to restore more efficient, natural, and pain-free movement.

5. Mind-Body Integration:

• Integration of Mind and Body: Somatic exercises promote the integration of mental, emotional, and physical aspects, emphasizing that changes in one aspect (e.g., physical tension) can influence others (e.g., emotions).

• Whole-Person Approach: Recognizing that the mind and body are interconnected systems, somatic practices consider the person as a whole entity rather than focusing solely on physical movements.

6. Self-Exploration and Empowerment:

• Self-Exploration: Practitioners are encouraged to explore their body's sensations and movements, fostering a sense of curiosity, self-discovery, and self-exploration.

• Empowerment: Somatic exercises empower individuals by providing tools for self-care, stress reduction, and improved well-being, allowing them to take an active role in their health.

7. Integration into Daily Life:

• Application Beyond Practice Sessions: Somatic principles extend beyond formal exercise sessions, encouraging practitioners to integrate mindful movement and body awareness into daily activities and routines.

By embodying these fundamental principles, somatic exercises offer a pathway for individuals to deepen their understanding of their bodies, promote relaxation, improve movement patterns, and cultivate a harmonious relationship between the mind and body, ultimately supporting holistic well-being.

THE IMPORTANCE OF MINDFULNESS AND BODY AWARENESS IN SOMATIC EXERCISES

Mindfulness and body awareness play pivotal roles in somatic exercises, forming the core foundation of these practices. Their importance lies in fostering a deeper connection between the mind and body, enhancing self-awareness, and facilitating holistic well-being. Here's why mindfulness and body awareness are crucial in somatic exercises:

1. Enhancing Internal Awareness:

• Mindfulness: Encourages practitioners to be fully present in the moment, observing bodily sensations, thoughts, and emotions without judgment. It enables individuals to become more attuned to their internal experiences during movement and stillness.

• Body Awareness: Focuses on perceiving and understanding internal bodily sensations, such as muscle tension, breathing patterns, and movement quality. This heightened awareness enables individuals to notice subtle changes and signals from their bodies.

2. Deepening the Mind-Body Connection:

• Mind-Body Integration: Mindfulness and body awareness foster a deeper connection between mental and physical states. Practitioners learn how thoughts, emotions, and physical sensations are interconnected, influencing one another.

• Embodied Cognition: By focusing attention on the body's sensations during movement, individuals develop a clearer understanding of how their thoughts and emotions manifest physically.

3. Cultivating Presence and Attention:

• Present-Moment Awareness: Mindfulness encourages practitioners to anchor their attention in the present moment, allowing them to experience movement and bodily sensations as they unfold in real-time.

• Focused Attention: Body awareness directs attention inward, facilitating a deeper exploration of bodily sensations, movements, and their relationship to mental states.

4. Stress Reduction and Relaxation:

• Stress Management: Mindfulness practices within somatic exercises promote relaxation responses in the body, reducing stress and promoting a sense of calmness and relaxation.

• Tension Release: Body awareness helps identify areas of muscular tension, enabling individuals to release chronic contractions and stress-related tension held within the body.

5. Improved Movement Quality and Efficiency:

• Movement Re-Education: Mindfulness and body awareness aid in re-educating movement patterns, enabling individuals to recognize and correct inefficient or habitual movements. This results in improved movement quality, coordination, and ease.

6. Self-Exploration and Empowerment:

• Self-Discovery: Practicing mindfulness and body awareness fosters self-exploration, allowing individuals to understand their body's needs, limitations, and potential for improvement.

• Empowerment: By being more attuned to their bodies, individuals feel empowered to take charge of their health and well-being, making informed choices about their movement and lifestyle.

7. Integration into Daily Life:

• Transferable Skills: Mindfulness and body awareness learned through somatic exercises can be applied beyond formal practice sessions, enriching daily life by promoting a more mindful approach to movement, stress management, and emotional regulation.

In essence, mindfulness and body awareness are essential components of somatic exercises, providing a pathway to deeper self-awareness, stress reduction, improved movement patterns, and ultimately supporting a more integrated and holistic sense of well-being.

THE SIGNIFICANCE OF BREATHING TECHNIQUES IN ENHANCING BODY AWARENESS.

Breathing techniques hold significant importance in enhancing body awareness within somatic practices. They serve as a gateway to deeper self-awareness, fostering a connection between the mind and body. Here's why breathing techniques are significant for enhancing body awareness:

1. Anchoring Attention:

• Focus Point: Utilizing specific breathing techniques provides a focal point for attention during somatic exercises. It directs attention inward, anchoring practitioners in the present moment and their bodily experiences.

2. Awareness of Body Sensations:

• Sensory Awareness: Breathing techniques encourage individuals to notice how different breathing patterns affect various body sensations, such as expansion and contraction of the chest, movement in the abdomen, or subtle changes in muscle tension.

• Connection to Body: Conscious breathing helps individuals perceive the intimate connection between their breath and bodily responses, heightening overall body awareness.

3. Regulation of Physical State:

• Stress Response: Controlled breathing aids in activating the body's relaxation response, reducing stress levels, and promoting a sense of calmness. This allows practitioners to observe how breathing influences their physiological state, emphasizing the mind-body connection.

• Muscle Tension: Deep, intentional breathing can assist in releasing muscular tension, promoting relaxation, and facilitating a clearer understanding of the body's response to different breathing patterns.

4. Mindful Movement and Posture:

• Support for Movement: Breath awareness complements movement, guiding practitioners to synchronize their breath with specific movements. This synchronization enhances movement quality, coordination, and posture, leading to a more integrated mind-body experience.

• Alignment and Awareness: Focusing on breath during movement encourages alignment awareness, allowing individuals to notice how their breath influences their body's alignment and posture.

5. Emotional Regulation:

• Emotional Connection: Conscious breathing techniques facilitate the regulation of emotions by promoting a sense of grounding and stability. It encourages practitioners to observe how breathing affects their emotional state, promoting emotional self-awareness.

6. Integration into Daily Life:

• Transferable Skill: Learning breath awareness and control within somatic exercises offers a skill applicable beyond formal practice sessions. Practitioners can use these techniques in daily life for stress management, relaxation, and emotional regulation.

7. Deepening Mind-Body Connection:

• Integration of Mind and Body: Through conscious breathing, individuals deepen their understanding of how mental states, emotions, and physical sensations are interconnected. This fosters a deeper mind-body connection and a sense of wholeness.

In summary, breathing techniques are pivotal in enhancing body awareness within somatic exercises. They serve as a gateway to heightened sensory perception, stress reduction, improved movement quality, emotional regulation, and an integrated mind-body experience, ultimately promoting a deeper understanding of oneself and the interconnectedness of the mind and body.

HOW TO SET UP A COMFORTABLE AND qUIET SPACE FOR PRACTICE

Creating a comfortable and quiet space for somatic exercise practice can significantly enhance your experience and focus. Here are steps to set up such a space:

1. Choose a Suitable Location:

• Space Availability: Select a room or area with enough space to move comfortably without obstacles or restrictions.

• Natural Light: If possible, opt for a space with natural light or adequate artificial lighting to create a pleasant atmosphere.

2. Clear the Space:

• Remove Clutter: Clear the area of unnecessary items, furniture, or clutter to create an open and unobstructed practice area.

• Safety Considerations: Ensure the space is safe for movement without any tripping hazards.

3. Comfortable Flooring:

• Yoga Mat or Soft Surface: Use a yoga mat, exercise mat, or a comfortable rug to provide a supportive and cushioned surface for lying down or sitting during exercises.

• Optional Props: Consider having additional props such as pillows, bolsters, or blankets for added comfort or support during relaxation exercises.

4. Quiet and Calm Environment:

• Noise Reduction: Choose a quiet environment, away from distractions or loud noises. Close doors or windows to minimize external disturbances.

• Background Music or Silence: Decide if you prefer practicing in silence or with calming background music to enhance relaxation. If using music, select soothing, instrumental tracks at a low volume.

5. Temperature and Ventilation:

• Comfortable Temperature: Ensure the room is at a comfortable temperature, neither too hot nor too cold, to facilitate relaxed movement.

• Ventilation: Maintain adequate airflow or ventilation to keep the space fresh and conducive to deep breathing.

6. Personalization and Ambiance:

• Aesthetics: Add personal touches such as plants, artwork, or decor that promote a sense of calmness and relaxation.

• Aromatherapy: Consider using essential oils or candles with calming scents to create a soothing ambiance (if preferred and suitable for the practice area).

7. Technology and Distractions:

• Minimize Distractions: Turn off or silence electronic devices to minimize distractions and interruptions during your practice.

• Useful Tools: If using instructional videos or guided practices, set up the necessary technology or equipment beforehand.

8. Personal Comfort:

• Appropriate Attire: Wear comfortable clothing that allows for unrestricted movement and promotes relaxation.

• Hydration: Keep a water bottle nearby to stay hydrated during and after your practice.

9. Mindful Intention:

• Setting Intentions: Before beginning your practice, take a moment to set an intention or focus for your session. This could be relaxation, increased body awareness, stress reduction, or any other goal you wish to achieve.

10. Regular Maintenance:

• Regular Cleaning: Maintain the cleanliness and tidiness of your practice space to ensure a welcoming environment for future sessions.

By following these steps, you can create a peaceful and inviting space conducive to somatic exercises, allowing you to immerse yourself fully in your practice and reap the benefits of mindful movement and relaxation.

THE IMPORTANCE OF RELAXATION

Relaxation holds immense importance for overall well-being and is a key component of somatic exercises. Here are the reasons why relaxation is crucial:

1. Stress Reduction:

• Stress Management: Relaxation techniques are powerful tools for reducing stress by activating the body's relaxation response. This helps lower cortisol levels, easing the body and mind from the effects of chronic stress.

2. Physical Health Benefits:

• Muscle Tension Release: Relaxation facilitates the release of muscular tension and stiffness, reducing physical discomfort and promoting better posture and flexibility.

• Lower Blood Pressure: Deep relaxation techniques contribute to lowering blood pressure and reducing the risk of cardiovascular issues.

3. Mental and Emotional Well-being:

• Calming the Mind: Relaxation practices calm the mind, reducing racing thoughts, anxiety, and feelings of overwhelm.

• Emotional Regulation: They promote emotional stability and resilience by allowing individuals to experience and manage their emotions more effectively.

4. Improved Sleep Quality:

• Better Sleep: Relaxation techniques aid in preparing the body and mind for sleep, improving sleep quality and duration. Quality sleep is crucial for overall health and well-being.

5. Enhanced Focus and Concentration:

• Mental Clarity: Relaxation fosters mental clarity, sharpens focus, and improves cognitive function. It can help individuals think more clearly and make decisions more effectively.

6. Pain Management:

• Pain Relief: Relaxation practices are often used as complementary approaches to manage pain, providing relief from chronic pain conditions by reducing muscle tension and promoting a sense of comfort.

7. Mind-Body Connection:

• Deepening Awareness: Relaxation techniques deepen the mind-body connection, allowing individuals to become more aware of bodily sensations, emotions, and how they are interconnected.

• Integration: They support the integration of physical, mental, and emotional aspects, fostering a more holistic approach to health and well-being.

8. Emotional Resilience:

• Strengthening Resilience: Regular relaxation practices contribute to building emotional resilience, helping individuals cope with life's challenges more effectively.

9. Overall Well-being and Quality of Life:

• Enhanced Quality of Life: By reducing stress, promoting relaxation, and supporting mental and physical health, relaxation significantly contributes to an improved overall quality of life.

10. Self-Care and Self-Awareness:

• Self-Care Practice: Relaxation techniques serve as a form of self-care, allowing individuals to prioritize their well-being and recharge themselves mentally and physically.

• Heightened Self-Awareness: Through relaxation practices, individuals gain a deeper understanding of their body's needs, stressors, and emotional responses, fostering greater self-awareness.

Incorporating relaxation into daily life, whether through mindfulness practices, deep breathing, meditation, or other relaxation techniques, is crucial for maintaining optimal health, managing stress, and fostering a balanced and harmonious mind-body connection.

CHAPTER TWO

THE DIFFERENT SOMATIC PRACTICES

Somatic practices encompass various mindful movement techniques that focus on integrating the mind, body, and breath to enhance body awareness, movement efficiency, and overall well-being. Here are explanations of different somatic practices:

1. Hanna Somatics:

• Developed by Thomas Hanna, Hanna Somatics emphasizes "pandiculation" – a combination of conscious movement and self-induced stretching to release chronic muscle tension.

• It aims to re-educate the neuromuscular system, improving posture, flexibility, and reducing pain by addressing sensory-motor amnesia.

2. Feldenkrais Method:

• Created by Moshe Feldenkrais, this method focuses on improving movement patterns and increasing awareness through gentle, mindful movements.

• It emphasizes learning through exploration, helping individuals reorganize movements to improve flexibility, coordination, and overall functioning.

3. Alexander Technique:

• The Alexander Technique aims to improve postural habits and movement by retraining the body to move with ease and efficiency.

• It focuses on releasing tension, improving posture, and developing body awareness to prevent unnecessary strain and promote graceful movement.

4. Body-Mind Centering (BMC):

• BMC involves embodying anatomical and developmental principles, exploring movement through the body's systems and tissues.

• It utilizes movement, touch, and imagery to explore bodily experiences, enhance self-awareness, and promote healing and personal growth.

5. Laban Movement Analysis:

• Developed by Rudolf Laban, this practice involves analyzing and understanding movement patterns, effort qualities, and space.

• It focuses on understanding how individuals move in space, providing insights into expressive movement and non-verbal communication.

6. Somatic Yoga:

• Combining traditional yoga practices with somatic principles, somatic yoga emphasizes internal body awareness, mindful movement, and breath-centered practices.

• It integrates elements of Feldenkrais, Alexander Technique, and other somatic practices into yoga postures and sequences.

7. Body-Mindfulness Practices:

• These practices involve cultivating mindfulness in movement, integrating meditation techniques into physical activities like walking, tai chi, or Qigong.

• The emphasis is on being fully present in each movement, fostering a deep mind-body connection and enhancing overall awareness.

Each somatic practice offers unique approaches to enhance body-mind connection, movement efficiency, and well-being. While they may differ in techniques and philosophies, their common goal is to help individuals improve movement patterns, reduce tension, and cultivate a deeper understanding of their bodies for overall health and vitality.

Hanna Somatics, developed by Thomas Hanna, is a method focused on improving body awareness, movement, and reducing chronic muscle tension through a process known as "pandiculation." This technique aims to re-educate the neuromuscular system to alleviate pain, restore movement patterns, and enhance flexibility.

Principles of Hanna Somatics:

• Sensory-Motor Amnesia (SMA):

Hanna Somatics addresses Sensory-Motor Amnesia, a condition where muscles become habitually contracted due to stress, injuries, or repetitive movements. This amnesia leads to reduced awareness and control over muscles.

• Pandiculation:

The core principle involves "pandiculation," a three-step process resembling the natural movement of animals upon waking. It includes voluntary contraction, release, and relaxation of specific muscles or muscle groups.

Key Components of Hanna Somatics:

• Education and Awareness: Hanna Somatics focuses on educating individuals about their habitual movement patterns and facilitating awareness of muscle tension through guided movement sequences.

• Gentle Movements and Repetition: Practitioners perform slow, gentle movements, encouraging the brain to re-establish proper muscle control. These movements are repeated to reinforce new neuromuscular patterns.

• Mind-Body Connection: Emphasizes the connection between the mind and body, using movement, breath, and conscious awareness to facilitate the release of chronic muscular tension.

Practice of Hanna Somatics:

• Guided Sessions: Typically, Hanna Somatics sessions involve guided movements performed slowly and mindfully under the instruction of a trained practitioner.

• Pandiculation Exercises: Practitioners guide individuals through specific pandiculation exercises, focusing on contracting and releasing targeted muscles to reset their resting lengths.

• Re-Educating Movement Patterns: By re-educating the nervous system, Hanna Somatics aims to restore natural movement patterns, reduce muscular tension, and alleviate pain caused by chronic muscular contraction.

• Daily Practice: Practitioners often encourage daily practice of gentle movements and pandiculation exercises at home to reinforce learning and facilitate long-term changes in muscle function and awareness.

Benefits of Hanna Somatics:

• Improved Flexibility and Movement: Releases chronic muscle tension, enhances flexibility, and restores natural movement patterns.

• Pain Relief: Alleviates pain caused by habitual muscle contraction and restores balance to the muscular system.

• Enhanced Body Awareness: Cultivates a deeper mind-body connection, promoting increased self-awareness and control over muscular tension.

Hanna Somatics offers a holistic approach to reprogramming the neuromuscular system, promoting relaxation, movement efficiency, and overall well-being by addressing Sensory-Motor Amnesia and chronic muscular tension through mindful movement practices.

THE FELDENKRAIS METHOD

The Feldenkrais Method, developed by Dr. Moshe Feldenkrais, is an educational system that explores movement, awareness, and learning to enhance physical and mental functioning. It's based on the principle that improving one's movement patterns and body awareness can lead to improvements in overall well-being. Here are the key aspects of the Feldenkrais Method:

• Awareness Through Movement (ATM):

Uses gentle movements and guided attention to increase self-awareness and explore movement possibilities. Practitioners are guided verbally through sequences of movements to discover new, more efficient ways of moving.

• Functional Integration (FI):

Involves one-on-one sessions with a certified practitioner who uses gentle touch, manipulation, and movement to address individual needs and improve movement patterns.

Key Components of the Feldenkrais Method:

• Gentle Movements: Focuses on slow, gentle movements that are easily accessible to individuals of all ages and physical abilities. Movements are designed to be comfortable and safe.

• Variation and Exploration: Emphasizes exploring a wide range of movements and variations, encouraging curiosity and discovery to improve movement quality and efficiency.

• Mind-Body Connection: Encourages awareness of habitual movement patterns, allowing individuals to explore new possibilities and refine their movements, fostering a deeper mind-body connection.

• Neuroplasticity and Learning: Capitalizes on the brain's ability to change and learn (neuroplasticity) by providing novel movement experiences to create new neural pathways and improve movement function.

Practice of the Feldenkrais Method:

• Awareness Through Movement (ATM) Classes: Group classes led by Feldenkrais practitioners involve verbally guided movement sequences. Participants explore movements while lying, sitting, or standing, focusing on refining coordination, flexibility, and relaxation.

• Functional Integration (FI) Sessions: Individual sessions conducted by a certified practitioner who provides personalized, hands-on guidance and gentle manipulations to address specific movement issues or support personal goals.

• Mindful Exploration: Emphasizes mindful exploration of movement, encouraging individuals to pay attention to sensations, habits, and limitations without judgment to facilitate learning and improvement.

Benefits of the Feldenkrais Method:

• Improved Movement Efficiency: Enhances movement quality, flexibility, coordination, and posture by exploring new movement patterns.

• Pain Relief: Helps reduce chronic pain by addressing movement imbalances and tension.

• Enhanced Body Awareness: Cultivates a heightened awareness of movement habits and encourages mindful exploration, leading to improved self-awareness and control.

The Feldenkrais Method offers a gentle, non-invasive approach to improve movement patterns and body awareness, promoting holistic well-being by focusing on individual learning and exploration. Through gentle movements and mindful awareness, individuals can discover new possibilities for movement and function in everyday activities.

THE ALEXANDER TECHNIQUE

The Alexander Technique, developed by F. Matthias Alexander, is an educational method aimed at improving movement coordination, posture, and overall well-being by retraining habitual patterns of movement and posture. It focuses on increasing self-awareness to bring about conscious control of one's movements and reactions. Here are the key components and principles of the Alexander Technique:

Principles of the Alexander Technique:

• Primary Control: Emphasizes the relationship between the head, neck, and back to achieve the "primary control" – a state where the head leads and the body follows in a coordinated, poised manner.

• Body Awareness and Inhibition: Encourages increased body awareness and the ability to "inhibit" or pause habitual responses, allowing individuals to avoid unnecessary tension or effort.

• Direction and Thought Process: Focuses on directing one's thoughts to influence movement, promoting mindful intention and conscious control over actions.

Key Components of the Alexander Technique:

• Postural Realignment: Addresses imbalances in posture and movement by identifying and correcting habits that interfere with natural alignment and coordination.

• Body Mapping and Kinesthetic Awareness: Educates individuals about their body's anatomical structure and movement, enhancing kinesthetic awareness for better movement efficiency.

• Mind-Body Integration: Promotes a holistic approach to movement and well-being, integrating the mind and body to improve overall functioning.

• Re-Education of Movement Patterns: Helps individuals unlearn harmful movement habits and re-educate themselves to move with greater ease, balance, and coordination.

• Individual Lessons (Hands-on Work): Conducted by certified Alexander Technique teachers, these one-on-one sessions involve gentle touch, verbal guidance, and hands-on work to help students recognize and release muscular tension, improve posture, and enhance movement coordination.

• Group Classes: Group sessions or workshops may focus on specific activities such as walking, sitting, or speaking to apply the principles of the Alexander Technique to everyday movements.

• Mindful Movement and Awareness: Practitioners are guided to perform simple movements with heightened awareness, observing and adjusting their habits to promote efficient, effortless movement.

Benefits of the Alexander Technique:

• Improved Posture and Alignment: Enhances overall posture, alignment, and coordination by addressing habitual movement patterns.

• Reduced Muscular Tension: Helps alleviate muscular tension, allowing for freer movement and reduced strain on the body.

• Enhanced Mind-Body Connection: Develops greater awareness and conscious control over movement, fostering a deeper mind-body connection.

The Alexander Technique offers a practical approach to relearning movement habits and improving overall functioning by promoting self-awareness, conscious movement, and improved coordination, ultimately leading to greater ease and efficiency in everyday activities.

BODY-MIND CENTERING

Body-Mind Centering (BMC), developed by Bonnie Bainbridge Cohen, is an embodied approach to movement, body awareness, and somatic education. It integrates principles from developmental movement, body systems, and embodied anatomy to explore the body's intelligence and enhance self-awareness. Here are the key components and principles of Body-Mind Centering:

Principles of Body-Mind Centering:

• Embodied Anatomy: Focuses on experiential anatomy, using movement, touch, and imagery to explore the body's structure, systems, and tissues from the inside out.

• Developmental Movement Patterns: Draws on early developmental movement patterns to understand how movement develops from infancy, emphasizing the role of these patterns in adult movement and function.

• Body Systems and Tissues: Studies the body's various systems (nervous, muscular, skeletal, etc.) and tissues (organs, fluids, cells) to understand their role in movement, perception, and overall well-being.

• Experiential Learning: Emphasizes learning through embodied experience, using guided movement, touch, and exploration to deepen self-awareness and understanding of the body.

• Hands-On Work: Practitioners may use hands-on techniques to facilitate movement, offer support, or guide individuals through somatic experiences, fostering a deeper connection with one's body.

• Movement and Expression: Encourages exploration of movement patterns, gestures, and expression to understand the body's expressive capabilities and improve movement quality.

• Mind-Body Integration: Integrates mental, emotional, and physical aspects to promote a holistic understanding of the body-mind connection.

• Experiential Workshops and Classes: Offers workshops, classes, and training programs that involve guided movement explorations, hands-on work, and discussions to deepen understanding of the body's systems and movements.

• Movement Repatterning: Practitioners guide individuals through movement sequences or exercises designed to explore and re-pattern habitual movement, facilitating greater freedom and efficiency.

• Embodied Anatomy Study: Involves experiential study of anatomical structures and body systems through touch, visualization, and movement to deepen understanding beyond traditional anatomical study.

Benefits of Body-Mind Centering:

• Improved Body Awareness: Enhances body awareness, sensory perception, and proprioception.

• Enhanced Movement Quality: Improves movement efficiency, coordination, and expression through re-patterning of movement habits.

• Holistic Well-Being: Integrates mental, emotional, and physical aspects, promoting overall well-being and self-discovery.

Body-Mind Centering offers a comprehensive approach to somatic education, integrating movement, anatomy, and embodiment practices to deepen self-awareness, enhance movement potential, and foster a deeper connection with the body-mind system.

Laban Movement Analysis (LMA) is a comprehensive framework developed by Rudolf Laban, a movement theorist and choreographer, to analyze and understand human movement. It provides a systematic approach to observing, describing, and interpreting movement patterns, qualities, and dynamics. LMA encompasses various components to analyze movement, including:

Components of Laban Movement Analysis:

• Body: LMA considers how the body moves in space and includes observing body parts, their relationships, and their interactions during movement.

• Effort: Analyzes movement qualities, such as time, weight, space, and flow, to understand the dynamics and expressive qualities of movement.

• Shape: Focuses on the forms and patterns created by the body during movement, considering both static and changing shapes.

• Space: Explores movement in relation to space, including the direction, level, size, and pathways of movement.

• Effort-Shape Framework: Describes movement qualities based on four effort elements: Weight, Time, Space, and Flow. These elements combine to create eight effort actions, each with specific characteristics.

• Motives and Drives: Identifies inner impulses or motives driving movement choices, considering both conscious and unconscious aspects of movement behavior.

• Phrasing and Dynamics: Analyzes movement sequences, rhythms, and dynamics to understand the timing, pacing, and energy of movement patterns.

• Qualities of Movement: Classifies movement qualities based on Laban's effort factors, describing movements as either strong or light, direct or indirect, bound or free, and sustained or sudden.

Practice and Application of Laban Movement Analysis:

• Observation and Description: LMA involves observing, describing, and documenting movement patterns and qualities using Laban's terminology and frameworks.

• Choreography and Performance: Applied in dance, theater, and performance arts to create and analyze movement sequences, develop characters, or explore choreographic elements.

• Therapeutic and Educational Settings: Utilized in movement therapy, somatic practices, and educational settings to enhance body awareness, movement potential, and expressiveness.

• Training and Analysis: Offers training programs and workshops for practitioners, performers, educators, and therapists to deepen their understanding and application of LMA.

Benefits of Laban Movement Analysis:

• Enhanced Movement Awareness: Improves understanding of movement dynamics, qualities, and expressive potential.

• Facilitates Creativity: Provides a framework for creating, analyzing, and understanding movement in various artistic and therapeutic contexts.

• Deepens Body-Mind Connection: Enhances awareness of the relationship between movement, emotion, and expression.

Laban Movement Analysis serves as a valuable tool for analyzing and understanding movement in various contexts, offering insights into movement qualities, patterns, and dynamics to enhance creativity, expressiveness, and body awareness.

Somatic Yoga combines principles from somatic practices, such as Body-Mind Centering, Feldenkrais Method, and Alexander Technique, with traditional yoga practices to enhance body awareness, movement quality, and overall well-being. It emphasizes internal body awareness, mindful movement, and breath-centered practices. Here are the key components and principles of Somatic Yoga:

Principles of Somatic Yoga:

• Body Awareness and Mindfulness: Emphasizes deepening awareness of bodily sensations, movements, and breath to foster a greater mind-body connection.

• Gentle Exploration and Movement: Focuses on slow, mindful movements to explore and re-pattern habitual movement habits, encouraging ease and efficiency in movement.

• Breath-Centered Practices: Integrates breath awareness and conscious breathing techniques to facilitate relaxation, release tension, and deepen the mind-body connection.

Key Components of Somatic Yoga:

• Somatic Movement Exploration: Incorporates exploratory movements inspired by somatic practices to deepen body awareness, improve movement quality, and release muscular tension.

• Mindful Asana Practice: Integrates traditional yoga postures (asanas) with somatic principles, focusing on slow, deliberate movements and mindful alignment to enhance body awareness.

• Breathwork and Relaxation: Incorporates breath-centered practices, such as pranayama and relaxation techniques, to promote relaxation, stress reduction, and deepen the mind-body connection.

Practice of Somatic Yoga:

• Mindful Movement Sequences: Involves slow and deliberate movement sequences that focus on internal body sensations, allowing practitioners to explore movement patterns with mindfulness.

• Breath-Centered Asana Practice: Practitioners engage in yoga postures with a focus on breath awareness, emphasizing smooth, conscious breaths synchronized with movement.

• Somatic Awareness and Release: Utilizes guided explorations and somatic movement practices to release tension, improve flexibility, and enhance body awareness.

Benefits of Somatic Yoga:

• Enhanced Body Awareness: Promotes a deeper understanding of the body's sensations, movements, and patterns.

• Improved Movement Quality: Encourages ease, efficiency, and fluidity in movement by re-patterning habitual movement habits.

• Stress Reduction and Relaxation: Integrates breathwork and relaxation techniques for relaxation, stress relief, and enhanced well-being.

Somatic Yoga offers a holistic approach to yoga practice, integrating somatic principles to deepen body awareness, enhance movement quality, and promote relaxation. By combining mindful movement, breath awareness, and somatic exploration, practitioners can experience greater ease, presence, and connection within their yoga practice and daily life.

BODY-MINDFULNESS PRACTICE

Body-mindfulness practice involves cultivating present-moment awareness and a deeper connection between the mind and body during various activities or movements. Rooted in mindfulness and somatic principles, it emphasizes bringing attention to bodily sensations, movements, and breath, fostering a heightened sense of awareness and presence. Here's a detailed exploration of body-mindfulness practice:

• Present-Moment Awareness: Emphasizes focusing attention on the present moment, observing bodily sensations, movements, and the surrounding environment without judgment.

• Mind-Body Connection: Cultivates an awareness of the interplay between thoughts, emotions, bodily sensations, and movements, recognizing their interconnectedness.

• Embodied Mindfulness: Integrates mindfulness practices with somatic principles, emphasizing awareness of bodily sensations and movements as a pathway to mindfulness.

Key Components of Body-Mindfulness Practice:

• Breath Awareness: Utilizes the breath as an anchor for mindfulness, directing attention to the sensations of breathing to ground oneself in the present moment.

• Somatic Exploration: Encourages exploratory movement practices, such as gentle stretches or body scans, to deepen awareness of bodily sensations and movement patterns.

• Mindful Movement: Applies mindfulness to movement activities, such as walking, yoga, or tai chi, focusing on the sensations and quality of movement.

• Body Scan and Relaxation: Involves a guided practice where attention is systematically directed through different parts of the body, promoting relaxation and heightened awareness.

Practice of Body-Mindfulness:

• Breath-Centered Practices: Engages in breath-focused meditation or pranayama exercises to anchor attention and cultivate present-moment awareness.

• Mindful Movement Activities: Participates in movement practices mindfully, paying attention to the sensations, breath, and movements during activities like walking, yoga, or qigong.

• Somatic Explorations: Engages in somatic practices or body scans to deepen awareness of bodily sensations, tensions, and movement possibilities.

• Everyday Mindfulness: Applies mindfulness to daily activities like eating, washing dishes, or sitting, focusing attention on the sensations and movements involved.

Benefits of Body-Mindfulness Practice:

• Stress Reduction: Promotes relaxation and reduces stress by fostering a grounded presence in the current moment.

• Enhanced Body Awareness: Develops a deeper understanding of bodily sensations, movements, and postures.

• Improved Mind-Body Connection: Strengthens the connection between the mind and body, fostering overall well-being and mental clarity.

Body-mindfulness practice offers a pathway to cultivate presence, self-awareness, and a deeper connection with oneself through the integration of mindfulness with embodied experiences and movements. It facilitates a more embodied and mindful way of living, fostering a sense of ease, balance, and presence in everyday life.

HOW TO PREPARE THE BODY FOR SOMATIC EXERCISES.

Preparing the body for somatic exercises involves a mindful approach to gradually awaken and tune into bodily sensations, allowing for a smoother transition into movement and heightened body awareness. Here's a step-by-step guide to prepare the body for somatic exercises:

1. Mindfulness and Centering:

• Centering Practice: Begin by finding a quiet space where you can sit comfortably. Close your eyes, take a few deep breaths, and bring your awareness to the present moment. Center yourself by focusing on your breath and allowing any thoughts to pass without attachment.

2. Body Scan and Relaxation:

• Body Awareness: Perform a brief body scan, starting from your head and moving down to your toes. Notice any areas of tension or discomfort. Take a few moments to consciously release tension by intentionally relaxing those areas.

3. Gentle Movement and Warm-Up:

• Slow Movement: Engage in slow, gentle movements to awaken the body gradually. Simple movements like shoulder rolls, neck stretches, gentle twists, or waist rotations can help loosen up the muscles and joints.

• Joint Mobilization: Perform gentle joint movements, such as wrist circles, ankle rotations, or knee bends, to improve joint mobility and prepare them for more extensive movement.

4. Breath Awareness:

• Breathing Exercises: Practice deep breathing exercises to further relax the body and bring attention to the breath. Inhale deeply through your nose, expanding your abdomen, and exhale slowly through your mouth, releasing any tension.

5. Somatic Exercises Preparation:

• Sensory Preparation: Spend a few moments focusing on the sensations in your body. Notice your posture, any areas of tightness, or areas that feel relaxed. This prepares your mind to be more attuned to bodily sensations during the exercises.

• Intentions Setting: Set intentions for your somatic practice. Whether it's increasing body awareness, releasing tension, or improving movement patterns, clarify your goals for the session.

6. Visualization and Mental Readiness:

• Visualize Movement: Visualize yourself performing the upcoming somatic exercises. Mentally prepare for the movements you are about to engage in, envisioning fluid and mindful movements.

• Cultivate Openness: Maintain an open and curious mindset, allowing yourself to explore sensations and movements without judgment or expectation.

7. Gradual Progression:

• Start Slowly: When beginning somatic exercises, start with simpler movements or exercises that feel comfortable and gradually progress to more challenging or complex movements.

• Listen to Your Body: Pay close attention to your body's responses and limitations. If you experience discomfort or pain, ease off or modify the movement accordingly.

8. Hydration and Comfort:

• Stay Hydrated: Ensure you are adequately hydrated before starting your practice session. Have water nearby to sip during breaks if needed.

• Comfortable Attire: Wear comfortable clothing that allows for unrestricted movement and promotes relaxation.

By following these steps, you can prepare your body effectively for somatic exercises, fostering a mindful and gentle approach that prioritizes body awareness, relaxation, and a gradual progression into movement practices.

IMPORTANCE OF COMFORTABLE CLOTHING

Comfortable clothing plays a crucial role in enhancing the effectiveness and comfort of various activities, including somatic exercises. Here's why comfortable attire is important:

• Freedom of Movement: Loose-fitting or stretchable clothing allows for unrestricted movement during exercises, enabling you to perform various somatic movements without constraints.

• Enhanced Body Sensation: Comfortable clothing that doesn't constrict the body facilitates better awareness of bodily sensations, helping you notice subtle changes or tensions during movements.

• Comfortable Temperature: Appropriate clothing helps regulate body temperature during exercises. Breathable fabrics or moisture-wicking materials can keep you comfortable by allowing airflow and preventing excessive sweating.

• Mindful Practice: Wearing comfortable clothing promotes a sense of ease and relaxation, allowing you to focus on the exercises and the sensations within your body without distractions from uncomfortable attire.

• Safety Consideration: Ill-fitting or restrictive clothing may pose safety risks during movement-based exercises. Comfortable attire reduces the risk of accidents or strains caused by clothing restrictions.

• Positive Mindset: Feeling comfortable and confident in your clothing can positively impact your mindset and motivation, encouraging a more enjoyable and consistent practice.

• Supportive Attire: Clothing that supports good posture and body alignment can complement somatic exercises by allowing you to maintain proper posture and movement patterns more easily.

• Personal Comfort: Wearing clothing that feels good and aligns with personal preferences contributes to a more positive exercise experience, encouraging regular participation in somatic practices.

Tips for Choosing Comfortable Clothing:

• Opt for stretchy, breathable fabrics like cotton, spandex, or moisture-wicking materials.

• Choose clothing that allows for ease of movement without being too tight or restrictive.

• Dress in layers to adjust to changes in temperature during exercise sessions.

• Consider wearing comfortable activewear or yoga attire that promotes flexibility and comfort.

• Prioritize comfort over fashion when selecting clothing for exercise sessions.

By selecting comfortable clothing tailored to support your movement and body awareness, you can enhance the effectiveness of somatic exercises, enabling a more enjoyable and focused practice session.

STEP-BY-STEP GUIDE ON HOW BEGINNERS CAN START WITH SOMATIC EXERCISES

Here's a step-by-step guide tailored for beginners to start with somatic exercises:

Step 1: Educate Yourself about Somatic Exercises

• Research and Learn: Explore resources about somatic exercises. Read books, watch instructional videos, or seek guidance from certified somatic practitioners to understand the principles and techniques.

Step 2: Prepare Your Space and Mind

• Create a Relaxing Space: Set up a quiet and comfortable area free from distractions for your practice sessions. Follow the guidelines to create a suitable space for somatic exercises.

• Mindfulness Practice: Begin each session with a few moments of mindfulness or deep breathing to center yourself and prepare your mind for the practice.

Step 3: Body Awareness and Warm-Up

• Body Scan: Perform a brief body scan, noticing areas of tension or discomfort. Relax those areas consciously.

• Gentle Warm-Up: Engage in slow and gentle movements to awaken the body. Start with simple stretches or joint movements to loosen up muscles and joints.

Step 4: Introduction to Somatic Exercises

• Basic Exercises: Start with foundational somatic exercises. These can include simple movements focusing on body awareness, such as pelvic tilts, gentle spinal movements, or mindful breathing exercises.

• Follow Guided Instructions: Use instructional resources or guided sessions tailored for beginners. Follow the step-by-step instructions provided by qualified instructors.

Step 5: Mindful Movement and Body Awareness

• Focus on Sensations: Pay attention to the sensations in your body as you perform each exercise. Notice areas of tension, movement quality, and how your body responds.

• Breathe Mindfully: Coordinate your breathing with movements. Inhale as you prepare for a movement and exhale as you release tension or complete the movement.

Step 6: Progression and Consistency

• Gradual Progression: Start with simpler exercises and gradually introduce more challenging movements or variations as you become more comfortable.

• Consistent Practice: Commit to regular practice sessions. Aim for shorter, frequent sessions initially, gradually increasing the duration as you progress.

Step 7: Self-Reflection and Adjustment

• Self-Reflection: After each session, reflect on your experience. Notice any changes in body sensations, areas of improvement, or challenges faced during the practice.

• Adjustment and Modification: Modify exercises if needed to suit your comfort level. Listen to your body and adjust movements or intensity to avoid discomfort or strain.

Step 8: Seek Guidance and Support

• Consult Professionals: Consider seeking guidance from certified somatic practitioners or attending introductory classes or workshops to deepen your understanding and practice.

• Join Communities: Engage with online forums or communities dedicated to somatic exercises. Share experiences, seek advice, and learn from others' journeys.

Step 9: Patience and Persistence

• Be Patient: Understand that progress takes time. Embrace the learning process and be patient with yourself as you explore somatic exercises.

• Stay Consistent: Maintain a consistent practice routine. Even small, regular efforts can yield significant results over time.

By following these steps and staying committed to your practice, you can gradually immerse yourself in the world of somatic exercises, enhancing body awareness, relaxation, and overall well-being. Remember to listen to your body, respect your limitations, and enjoy the journey of self-discovery and mindful movement.

CHAPTER THREE

BEGINNER-FRIENDLY EXERCISES THAT FOCUS ON BODY AWARENESS

Here are some beginner-friendly somatic exercises that focus on enhancing body awareness:

1. Mindful Breathing

Purpose: To center yourself, connect with your breath, and promote relaxation.

2. Pelvic Tilts

Purpose: To increase awareness of the pelvic region and release tension in the lower back.

3. Seated Spinal Twist

Purpose: To increase spinal mobility and promote body awareness along the spine.

4. Body Scan Meditation

Purpose: To increase overall body awareness and promote relaxation.

These beginner-friendly somatic exercises emphasize mindfulness, gentle movement, and body awareness, providing a foundation for increasing your sensitivity to bodily sensations and promoting relaxation. As you practice regularly, you'll gradually deepen your awareness and connection with your body.

BEGINNER-FRIENDLY EXERCISES THAT FOCUS ON GENTLE MOVEMENTS

Here are some gentle somatic exercises suitable for beginners that emphasize slow, mindful movements:

1. Somatic Shoulder Rolls

Purpose: To release tension in the shoulders and promote awareness of shoulder mobility.

2. Somatic Neck Stretches

Purpose: To increase mobility and release tension in the neck.

3. Somatic Side Bends

Purpose: To improve lateral mobility and release tension along the sides of the body.

4. Somatic Hip Circles

Purpose: To increase mobility and awareness in the hips and lower back.

5. Somatic Knee-to-Chest Stretch

Purpose: To gently stretch the lower back and increase flexibility.

These beginner-friendly somatic exercises emphasize slow, mindful movements to enhance body awareness, promote gentle stretching, and encourage relaxation. Practice at your own pace, paying attention to your body's feedback, and enjoy the benefits of mindful movement.

BEGINNER-FRIENDLY EXERCISES THAT FOCUS ON RELAXATION

Here are some beginner-friendly somatic exercises specifically designed to promote relaxation:

1. Full Body Relaxation Scan

Purpose: To relax the entire body and increase overall body awareness.

2. Progressive Muscle Relaxation

Purpose: To release tension in specific muscle groups through a progressive relaxation sequence.

3. Diaphragmatic Breathing

Purpose: To promote relaxation and activate the body's relaxation response.

4. Guided Visualization Meditation

Purpose: To induce a state of relaxation through mental imagery and visualization.

5. Body Swaying or Rocking

Purpose: To induce relaxation by promoting gentle, rhythmic movement.

These beginner-friendly somatic exercises emphasize relaxation techniques such as deep breathing, progressive muscle relaxation, visualization, and gentle movements to induce a state of calmness and relaxation. Practice these exercises regularly to experience increased relaxation and stress relief.

Here's a step-by-step guide to practicing mindful breathing:

Step-by-Step Guide to Mindful Breathing:

• Find a Comfortable Position: Sit in a comfortable chair or cross-legged on the floor. Ensure your spine is comfortably straight, shoulders relaxed, and hands resting gently on your lap or knees.

• Relaxation Posture: Close your eyes gently or keep them softly focused on a spot in front of you. Allow your facial muscles, jaw, and shoulders to relax.

• Connect with Your Breath: Begin by taking a few deep breaths, inhaling through your nose and exhaling through your mouth. Feel the sensations of the breath entering and leaving your body.

• Shift to Natural Breathing: Gradually transition to your natural breathing pattern, inhaling and exhaling through your nose. Notice the movement of your breath — how the air feels as it enters and exits your nostrils.

• Focus on the Breath: Direct your attention to the physical sensations associated with breathing. Feel the rise and fall of your abdomen or chest with each breath. Observe the pace, depth, and rhythm of your breath without trying to change it.

• Anchor Your Attention: Choose a specific area to focus on, such as the sensation of air passing through your nostrils, the rise and fall of your chest, or the gentle expansion and contraction of your abdomen.

• Stay Present: Your mind may wander — thoughts, distractions, or sensations might arise. Acknowledge these thoughts or distractions without judgment and gently guide your attention back to your chosen focal point — the sensation of breathing.

• Observe Without Judgment: Be an impartial observer of your breath. Notice the nuances of each inhale and exhale without labeling them as good or bad. Simply observe the experience.

• Practice Gratitude: If your mind wanders, gently guide it back to your breath, expressing gratitude for the opportunity to connect with your breath and be present in the moment.

• Continue for a Few Minutes: Engage in mindful breathing for a few minutes, gradually increasing the duration as you become more comfortable. Start with 5–10 minutes and extend the practice over time.

• Closure: To conclude, take a few deep breaths, gently wiggle your fingers and toes, and slowly open your eyes if they were closed.

Remember, the essence of mindful breathing is to cultivate a non-judgmental awareness of your breath and the present moment. With practice, mindful breathing can promote relaxation, reduce stress, and enhance your overall sense of well-being. Gradually integrating this practice into your daily routine can yield significant benefits over time.

When practicing mindful breathing, paying attention to posture, utilizing breathing cues, and maintaining awareness are crucial components for an effective and beneficial experience. Here's an explanation of each:

Posture:

• Alignment: Sit or stand in a posture that supports alertness and relaxation. Keep your spine comfortably straight, allowing the natural curves of your spine to be present. Avoid slouching or overarching your back.

• Relaxed Body: Relax your shoulders, allowing them to drop naturally away from your ears. Let your hands rest comfortably on your lap or knees. Loosen any tension in your facial muscles and jaw.

• Grounding: If sitting, place your feet flat on the floor. If standing, ensure a stable base by keeping your feet hip-width apart. Feel connected to the ground, fostering a sense of stability.

• Comfort: Find a position that is comfortable for you, allowing you to maintain the posture without strain throughout your practice session.

Breathing Cue:

• Natural Breathing: Begin with natural, unforced breathing. Inhale and exhale through your nose, allowing the breath to be smooth and relaxed.

• Focus Point: Choose a specific focus point for your breath — this could be the sensation of air passing through your nostrils, the rise and fall of your chest or abdomen, or the sound of your breath.

• Gentle Attention: Direct your attention to your chosen focus point, gently observing the breath without trying to control it. Let the breath flow naturally while maintaining awareness.

Awareness:

• Present Moment Awareness: Be fully present in the moment, observing the sensations of breathing as they occur without dwelling on the past or anticipating the future.

• Non-Judgmental Observation: Notice the breath and any arising thoughts, emotions, or distractions without judgment. Acknowledge them and gently guide your attention back to your breath.

• Open Awareness: Expand your awareness to encompass the entire body if possible. Notice any tension, discomfort, or areas of relaxation in your body as you breathe.

• Gratitude and Compassion: Cultivate an attitude of gratitude and compassion toward yourself as you practice mindful breathing, appreciating the opportunity to nurture your well-being.

By maintaining a mindful posture, utilizing breathing cues to focus attention, and cultivating a non-judgmental awareness of the present moment, you can deepen your practice of mindful breathing. These elements work together to facilitate relaxation, reduce stress, and enhance your overall sense of calm and presence. Regular practice can further strengthen these skills and benefits over time.

Pelvic tilts are simple yet effective exercises that can help increase awareness of your pelvic region and release tension in your lower back. Here's a step-by-step guide on how to perform pelvic tilts:

Pelvic Tilt Exercise:

Starting Position:

• Lie on your back on a comfortable surface, such as a yoga mat or carpeted floor.

• Bend your knees with feet flat on the floor, hip-width apart.

• Ensure your arms are relaxed by your sides, palms facing down.

Neutral Spine Position:

• In this position, your lower back has a natural curve with a small gap between your lower back and the floor.

• Engage your abdominal muscles slightly, but avoid pressing your lower back into the floor forcefully.

Performing the Pelvic Tilt:

• Inhale to prepare.

• As you exhale, gently tilt your pelvis backward by pressing your lower back into the floor.

• Feel your tailbone lifting slightly and your lower back flattening against the floor.

• Your abdominal muscles will naturally engage during this movement.

Hold the Tilt:

• Hold the position for a few seconds while maintaining a steady and controlled breath.

• Focus on the sensation of your pelvis tilting and the engagement of your abdominal muscles.

Return to Neutral Position:

• Inhale and gradually release the pelvic tilt, allowing your lower back to return to its neutral position.

• Feel the natural curve returning to your lower back as you release the tilt.

Repetition:

• Repeat the movement for several repetitions, coordinating the movement with your breath.

• Gradually increase the number of repetitions as you become more familiar with the exercise.

Mindful Awareness:

• Throughout the exercise, maintain awareness of the sensations in your lower back, pelvis, and abdomen.

• Be mindful of any tension or discomfort and adjust the movement if needed to avoid strain.

Relaxation:

• After completing the repetitions, relax in a comfortable position, taking a few deep breaths to allow your body to settle.

Tips:

• Perform the pelvic tilts slowly and gently, focusing on the quality of the movement rather than the quantity.

• Avoid overarching or forcing your lower back into the floor excessively.

• If you have any existing back issues or injuries, consult a healthcare professional before practicing pelvic tilts or any new exercise.

Pelvic tilts can be incorporated into your daily routine to promote greater awareness of your pelvic alignment and help alleviate tension in the lower back, contributing to better posture and overall body comfort.

When practicing pelvic tilts, focusing on posture, utilizing appropriate breathing cues, and maintaining awareness are essential for an effective and safe exercise experience. Here's an explanation of each aspect:

Posture:

• Supine Position: Begin by lying on your back (supine position) on a comfortable surface, such as a yoga mat or carpet.

• Neutral Spine: Maintain a neutral spine position, where there's a natural curve in your lower back with a small gap between the floor and your lower back. Avoid excessive arching or pressing the lower back forcefully into the floor.

• Relaxed Upper Body: Keep your arms relaxed by your sides, palms facing down, and shoulders comfortably resting on the ground.

• Feet Placement: Bend your knees and place your feet flat on the floor, hip-width apart, ensuring your feet are comfortable and grounded.

Breathing Cue:

• Inhalation and Exhalation: Sync your breath with the movement of the pelvic tilt.

• Exhale during Tilt: As you initiate the pelvic tilt by gently pressing your lower back into the floor, exhale slowly and steadily. This can help engage your core muscles and aid in relaxation.

• Inhale for Release: As you return to the neutral position, inhale gradually and allow your lower back to return to its natural curve.

Awareness:

• Pelvic Movement Awareness: Focus on the sensation of tilting your pelvis as you perform the exercise. Be aware of how your tailbone slightly lifts and your lower back flattens against the floor during the tilt.

• Abdominal Engagement: Notice the engagement of your abdominal muscles as you tilt your pelvis backward. This engagement supports the movement and stability.

• Body Sensations: Be mindful of any tension or discomfort during the exercise. If you feel strain or excessive discomfort, adjust the movement or range of motion to a more comfortable level.

• Quality over Quantity: Prioritize the quality of the movement over the number of repetitions. Perform the pelvic tilts slowly and with control, focusing on the sensation and engagement of the muscles involved.

• Relaxation and Release: After completing the repetitions, relax and breathe deeply for a moment, allowing your body to return to a neutral and relaxed state.

• If you have any existing back issues, injuries, or concerns, consult a healthcare professional or physical therapist before performing pelvic tilts or any new exercise.

By maintaining proper posture, syncing your breath with the movement, and fostering mindful awareness of sensations and muscle engagement, you can perform pelvic tilts effectively and safely, promoting greater pelvic awareness and potential relief from lower back discomfort.

Seated spinal twists are beneficial for increasing spinal mobility and promoting flexibility. Here's a step-by-step guide on how to perform a seated spinal twist:

Seated Spinal Twist Exercise:

Starting Position:

• Sit comfortably on the floor or on a chair with your spine tall and your shoulders relaxed.

• Extend your legs in front of you if seated on the floor or keep them bent if sitting on a chair.

• Ensure both feet are firmly grounded.

Inhale to Lengthen:

• Inhale deeply and lengthen your spine, imagining the crown of your head reaching toward the ceiling.

Twisting to One Side:

• Exhale and gently twist your upper body to one side, moving from your waist, not just your shoulders.

• Place your hand on the outside of the opposite knee or the armrest of the chair for support.

• Use your other hand behind you for additional support, placing it on the floor or the backrest of the chair.

Maintain Length in the Spine:

• With each inhale, lengthen your spine upward, maintaining the elongation.

• With each exhale, gently deepen the twist, ensuring it is comfortable and not forced.

Hold the Twist:

• Hold the twist for a few breaths, maintaining a steady and relaxed breath pattern.

• Feel the gentle rotation along your spine and the stretch through your torso.

Release and Switch Sides:

• Inhale as you gradually release the twist, returning your upper body to the center.

• Exhale and repeat the twisting motion in the opposite direction.

• Place your hand on the opposite knee or chair armrest, and the other hand for support behind you.

Mindful Breathing and Awareness:

• Throughout the exercise, maintain a steady and controlled breath, inhaling and exhaling smoothly.

• Pay attention to the sensations along your spine, noticing the gentle stretch and release as you twist.

Comfort and Modification:

• If you experience discomfort or strain, reduce the intensity of the twist or refrain from twisting as deeply.

• Adapt the movement to suit your comfort level, ensuring a gentle and controlled rotation.

Repetition and Closure:

• Repeat the twist on each side for several repetitions, alternating sides.

• After completing the twists, return to a neutral seated position and take a few deep breaths to relax.

Tips:

• Perform the seated spinal twist slowly and gently, focusing on maintaining proper form and alignment.

• Avoid forcing the twist beyond your comfortable range of motion.

• If seated on a chair, ensure the chair is stable and provides adequate support during the movement.

Seated spinal twists can help improve spinal flexibility and promote a sense of relaxation. Incorporate this exercise into your routine to enhance your overall mobility and comfort. If you have any existing back issues or concerns, consult a healthcare professional before performing spinal twist exercises.

POSTURE, BREATHING CUE AND AWARENESS WHEN PRACTICING SEATED SPINAL TWIST

Practicing a seated spinal twist involves maintaining proper posture, syncing your breath with the movement, and being aware of sensations throughout the exercise. Here's an explanation of each aspect:

Posture:

• Seated Position: Sit comfortably on the floor with your legs extended or on a chair with feet grounded, ensuring stability and comfort.

• Tall Spine: Lengthen your spine by sitting tall, imagining the crown of your head reaching upward toward the ceiling.

• Shoulder Relaxation: Keep your shoulders relaxed and away from your ears, allowing for ease of movement.

• Grounded Base: Ensure both feet are firmly planted on the floor. If sitting on the floor, cross-legged, maintain a stable and grounded base.

Breathing Cue:

• Inhalation and Exhalation: Sync your breath with the movement of the twist.

• Inhale for Lengthening: Inhale deeply to lengthen your spine and create space in your torso.

• Exhale for the Twist: Exhale slowly and steadily as you initiate the twist, using the exhale to deepen the movement.

Awareness:

• Initiating the Twist: Gently initiate the twist from your waist, not just your shoulders, gradually rotating your upper body to one side.

• Spinal Sensation: Focus on the sensations along your spine as you twist, feeling the gentle stretch and release in the muscles along the torso.

• Breath and Movement Synchronization: Maintain awareness of your breath throughout the twist, ensuring a steady and controlled breath pattern that complements the movement.

• Comfort and Adjustments: Be mindful of your body's limits and comfort. If you feel any discomfort or strain, ease out of the twist slightly or modify the movement to a more comfortable range.

• Opposite Side Twist: After holding the twist for a few breaths, gently return to the center with an inhale, then exhale and repeat the twist on the opposite side.

• Mindful Release: Gradually release the twist with control, allowing your torso to return to the center, and take a moment to feel the effects of the movement.

Safety Note:

• If you have any existing spinal issues or concerns, approach the seated spinal twist with caution and consider consulting a healthcare professional before performing the exercise.

By maintaining proper posture, synchronizing your breath with the movement, and fostering awareness of sensations, you can practice the seated spinal twist effectively and safely, enhancing spinal mobility and promoting a sense of relaxation.

STEP-BY-STEP GUIDE TO BODY SCAN MEDITATION

Body scan meditation is a mindfulness practice that involves systematically directing attention to different parts of the body, cultivating awareness and relaxation. Here's a step-by-step guide on how to practice body scan meditation:

Body Scan Meditation:

Comfortable Position:

• Find a comfortable position, either lying down on your back or sitting in a relaxed posture. Ensure you're in a quiet environment with minimal distractions.

Relaxation Preparation:

• Close your eyes gently if comfortable, or maintain a soft gaze.

• Take a few deep breaths to relax and center yourself. Inhale through your nose, exhale through your mouth, releasing tension with each breath.

Begin at the Feet:

• Direct your attention to your feet. Focus on the sensations in your toes, the soles of your feet, and the tops of your feet.

• Notice any sensations—warmth, tingling, pressure, or relaxation. Acknowledge them without judgment.

Progress through Each Body Part:

• Move your attention slowly upward, to your ankles, calves, knees, thighs, and hips, one part at a time.

• With each body part, take a moment to notice sensations, tensions, or relaxation present in that area.

Torso and Arms:

• Continue to the torso, noticing the sensations in your abdomen, lower back, upper back, chest, shoulders, and arms.

• Be aware of any areas of tightness, comfort, or release, allowing your breath to soften those areas.

Neck and Head:

• Move your attention to your neck, noticing any sensations in the front, sides, and back of your neck.

• Finally, focus on your head, including your facial muscles, jaw, and the crown of your head. Acknowledge any sensations present.

Observation without Judgment:

• Throughout the body scan, observe each body part without judging or trying to change anything. Simply notice what is present, accepting sensations as they are.

Gentle Breath Awareness:

• If your mind wanders, gently guide your attention back to the body part you're focusing on and reconnect with your breath.

• Use the breath as an anchor, allowing it to accompany your awareness of each body area.

Closure and Relaxation:

• After scanning the entire body, take a few moments to experience the sensations of your entire body as a whole, from head to toe.

• Gradually deepen your breaths, slowly wiggle your fingers and toes, and when you're ready, open your eyes if they were closed.

Tips:

• Practice the body scan meditation at your own pace, taking your time with each body part.

• If distractions arise, gently guide your attention back to the present moment and the area you're focusing on.

• Start with shorter sessions (5-10 minutes) and gradually extend the duration as you become more comfortable with the practice.

Body scan meditation can foster relaxation, increase body awareness, and promote a sense of mindfulness. Regular practice can help reduce stress and enhance overall well-being by cultivating a deeper connection with your body and sensations.

POSTURE, BREATHING CUE AND AWARENESS WHEN PRACTICING BODY SCAN MEDITATION

Practicing body scan meditation involves maintaining a relaxed posture, using the breath as a cue, and fostering awareness throughout the exercise. Here's a breakdown of each aspect:

Posture:

Comfortable Position:

• Find a comfortable position, either lying down on your back with legs extended or sitting in a relaxed posture on a chair or cushion.

• Ensure your body is supported and you can maintain the position without strain for the duration of the practice.

Relaxed Body:

• Allow your body to relax and settle into the chosen position.

• If lying down, keep your arms by your sides, palms facing up. If sitting, rest your hands comfortably on your lap or thighs.

Spinal Alignment:

• If sitting, ensure your spine is comfortably straight but not rigid, allowing for natural curves.

• If lying down, let your spine rest in its natural alignment, maintaining comfort.

Breathing Cue:

• Natural Breathing: Begin by taking a few deep, relaxing breaths to center yourself and establish a relaxed breathing pattern.

• Steady Breath Awareness: As you progress through the body scan, maintain a steady and natural breath, using it as an anchor to stay present.

• Gentle Breathing: Breathe naturally and gently, without forcing or controlling the breath. Let it flow comfortably in and out of your body.

Awareness:

• Body Part Focus: Start the body scan by directing your attention to one body part at a time, progressing systematically from feet to head or vice versa.

• Sensory Awareness: Focus on the sensations present in each body part—warmth, tingling, pressure, relaxation, or any other sensations.

• Non-Judgmental Observation: Observe each body part without judgment or the need to change anything. Accept the sensations as they are without evaluation.

• Mindful Attention: If distractions arise, gently guide your attention back to the body part you're focusing on and the sensations present there.

• Breath and Body Connection: Use your breath as a bridge to connect with each body part. Notice how the breath affects the sensations in each area.

Closure and Relaxation:

• Closing the Practice: After scanning the entire body, gradually bring your attention back to your entire body as a whole.

• Deepening Breath: Take a few deep breaths, gently wiggling your fingers and toes to reawaken your body.

• Transitioning Back: Slowly open your eyes if they were closed and allow yourself a moment to readjust before resuming any activities.

Tips:

• Approach the body scan meditation with a gentle and open attitude, allowing sensations to arise and fade without attachment.

• If your mind wanders, gently guide your focus back to the body part you're attending to and reconnect with your breath.

By maintaining a relaxed posture, using the breath as a guide, and fostering non-judgmental awareness, body scan meditation can deepen your connection with bodily sensations and promote a sense of relaxation and mindfulness.

STEP-BY-STEP GUIDE TO SOMATIC SHOULDER ROLLS

Somatic shoulder rolls are gentle exercises that can help release tension in the shoulders and promote relaxation. Here's a step-by-step guide on how to perform somatic shoulder rolls:

Somatic Shoulder Rolls Exercise:

• Comfortable Position: Stand or sit comfortably in a relaxed posture with your spine comfortably straight.

• Relaxation Preparation: Allow your arms to rest by your sides in a relaxed manner. Let your shoulders relax away from your ears.

• Starting Position: Inhale deeply to prepare, and as you exhale, gently lift your shoulders up toward your ears, creating tension in the shoulder muscles.

• Rolling Movement: As you continue exhaling, begin to roll your shoulders backward in a circular motion. Gradually move your shoulders away from your ears and down, focusing on the full rotation of the movement.

• Completing the Circle: Continue the circular motion until your shoulders have completed a full rotation. Feel the gentle stretch and release in the shoulder muscles as you perform the movement.

• Reverse Direction: Inhale as you lift your shoulders up again, this time rolling them forward in a circular motion. Complete a full circle, bringing your shoulders up toward the ears, forward, down, and back to the starting position.

• Mindful Breathing: Throughout the exercise, maintain a relaxed and steady breath. Inhale and exhale comfortably without strain.

• Awareness of Shoulder Movement: Focus on the sensations in your shoulders as you perform the rolling movement. Notice any areas of tension or relaxation.

• Quality of Movement: Perform the shoulder rolls slowly and mindfully, emphasizing the quality of the movement rather than speed. Ensure the movement is gentle and comfortable without causing any discomfort or strain.

• Repetition: Repeat the shoulder rolls for several repetitions, alternating between backward and forward rotations. Aim for a smooth and controlled motion with each repetition.

Tips:

• Start with a smaller range of motion if you're new to this exercise, gradually increasing the movement as your muscles loosen.

• Avoid tensing the neck or other areas of the body. Focus specifically on the movement in the shoulders.

• Perform this exercise at your own pace, allowing for a relaxing and enjoyable experience.

Somatic shoulder rolls can help alleviate shoulder tension and enhance mobility. Regular practice of this gentle exercise can contribute to increased relaxation and improved shoulder comfort.

When practicing somatic shoulder rolls, focusing on posture, syncing your breath with the movement, and maintaining awareness are essential for an effective and safe exercise. Here's an explanation of each aspect:

Posture:

• Relaxed Position: Stand or sit comfortably with a relaxed posture. Ensure your spine is comfortably straight but not rigid, allowing for natural alignment.

• Shoulder Relaxation: Allow your arms to hang naturally by your sides, and let your shoulders relax away from your ears. Ensure your body is comfortable and at ease, without unnecessary tension in the neck, shoulders, or back.

Breathing Cue:

• Natural Breathing Rhythm: Begin the exercise by taking a few deep, relaxing breaths to center yourself and establish a calm breathing pattern.

• Syncing Breath with Movement: Inhale deeply as you initiate the lifting of your shoulders toward your ears. Exhale gradually and steadily as you roll your shoulders backward or forward in a circular motion.

• Focused Attention on Shoulders: Direct your attention to the sensations in your shoulders as you perform the rolling movement. Notice how your shoulders move upward toward your ears, backward, downward, and forward in a circular pattern.

• Sensory Awareness: Be mindful of any areas of tension, discomfort, or relief in the shoulder muscles during the movement. Observe the changes in sensation as you perform the shoulder rolls, paying attention to any tightness or relaxation.

• Gentle and Controlled Movement: Perform the shoulder rolls slowly and gently, emphasizing smooth and controlled rotations. Avoid abrupt or jerky movements, allowing the shoulders to move in a relaxed and fluid manner.

• Breath and Body Connection: Use your breath as a guide to accompany the movement, maintaining a steady and calm breathing pattern throughout the exercise. Sync your awareness of the shoulder movement with the natural flow of your breath, promoting relaxation.

Tips:

• Maintain a relaxed and non-strained posture throughout the exercise, focusing specifically on the movement in the shoulders.

• Be mindful of your body's response, adjusting the range of motion or speed of the shoulder rolls to suit your comfort level.

• Perform the exercise at a pace that allows you to remain present and aware of the sensations in your shoulders.

By maintaining a relaxed posture, syncing breath with movement, and fostering sensory awareness, somatic shoulder rolls can help release tension in the shoulders and promote relaxation and comfort in this area.

STEP-BY-STEP GUIDE TO SOMATIC NECK STRETCHES

Somatic neck stretches are gentle exercises designed to alleviate tension and promote relaxation in the neck muscles. Here's a step-by-step guide on how to perform somatic neck stretches:

Somatic Neck Stretches:

• Comfortable Position: Sit or stand comfortably in a relaxed posture, ensuring your spine is comfortably straight.

• Relaxation Preparation: Allow your shoulders to relax, keeping them away from your ears. Find a quiet environment where you can perform the stretches without distractions.

• Starting Position: Begin by sitting tall or standing comfortably with a relaxed stance. Keep your chin parallel to the ground and your gaze forward.

• Chin Tuck Stretch: Inhale deeply to prepare. As you exhale, gently tuck your chin toward your chest, feeling a stretch along the back of your neck. Hold the stretch for a few seconds, maintaining a comfortable and relaxed breath.

• Ear to Shoulder Stretch (Right Side): Inhale deeply again. As you exhale, slowly tilt your right ear toward your right shoulder, feeling a gentle stretch along the left side of your neck. Avoid lifting your shoulder; keep it relaxed. Hold the stretch for a few seconds while breathing naturally and comfortably.

• Ear to Shoulder Stretch (Left Side): Inhale once more. Exhale and slowly tilt your left ear toward your left shoulder, feeling a gentle stretch along the right side of your neck. Maintain a relaxed breath and hold the stretch for a few seconds.

• Half Neck Rotation (Right Side): Inhale deeply to prepare. As you exhale, turn your head to the right, aiming to bring your chin towards your right shoulder. Feel a gentle stretch on the left side of your neck. Hold the position for a few seconds while maintaining relaxed breathing.

• Half Neck Rotation (Left Side): Inhale again. Exhale and turn your head to the left, aiming to bring your chin towards your left shoulder. Feel a gentle stretch on the right side of your neck. Hold the position for a few seconds while breathing comfortably.

• Mindful Awareness: Throughout the stretches, maintain awareness of the sensations in your neck, noticing any areas of tension or relaxation.

• Relaxation and Closure: After performing each stretch on both sides, return your head to a neutral position. Take a moment to relax, breathe deeply, and allow your neck muscles to release any remaining tension.

Tips:

• Perform the stretches slowly and gently, without forcing the movement or causing discomfort.

• Focus on the quality of the stretch rather than the intensity, allowing the muscles to relax gradually.

• If you have any neck issues or discomfort, perform the stretches within your comfort range or consult a healthcare professional for guidance.

Regular practice of somatic neck stretches can help reduce neck tension and enhance flexibility in the neck muscles, promoting a sense of relaxation and comfort in the neck area.

POSTURE, BREATHING CUE AND AWARENESS WHEN PRACTICING SOMATIC NECK STRETCHES

Practicing somatic neck stretches involves maintaining a relaxed posture, syncing your breath with the movement, and fostering awareness throughout the exercise. Here's an explanation of each aspect:

Posture:

• Comfortable Position: Sit or stand comfortably with a relaxed but upright posture. Ensure your spine is comfortably straight, allowing for natural alignment.

• Shoulder Relaxation: Keep your shoulders relaxed and away from your ears. Allow your arms to rest comfortably by your sides or on your lap.

• Neutral Head Position: Keep your head in a neutral position, with your chin parallel to the ground and your gaze straight ahead.

Breathing Cue:

• Natural Breathing Rhythm: Begin the stretches by taking a few deep, calming breaths to center yourself and establish a relaxed breathing pattern.

• Syncing Breath with Movement: Inhale deeply before initiating the stretch. Exhale slowly and steadily as you perform each stretch, allowing the exhalation to accompany the movement.

Awareness:

• Focused Attention on Neck Sensations: Direct your attention to the sensations in your neck as you perform each stretch. Notice the gentle stretching sensation along the sides and back of your neck during each movement.

• Sensory Awareness: Be mindful of any areas of tension, discomfort, or release in the neck muscles as you perform the stretches. Observe the changes in sensation with each movement, paying attention to the quality of the stretch.

• Gentle and Controlled Movement: Perform the stretches slowly and smoothly, emphasizing a gentle and controlled range of motion. Avoid jerky or abrupt movements, allowing the neck muscles to stretch gradually and comfortably.

• Breath and Body Connection: Use your breath as a guide to accompany the movement, ensuring a relaxed and steady breath pattern throughout the stretches. Sync your awareness of the neck movement with the natural rhythm of your breath, promoting relaxation.

Tips:

• Maintain a relaxed and non-strained posture throughout the stretches, focusing specifically on the movement in the neck.

• Be mindful of your body's response, adjusting the intensity or duration of the stretches to suit your comfort level.

• Perform the stretches at a pace that allows you to remain present and aware of the sensations in your neck.

By maintaining a relaxed posture, syncing breath with movement, and fostering sensory awareness, somatic neck stretches can help alleviate tension and promote relaxation in the neck muscles.

STEP-BY-STEP GUIDE TO SOMATIC SIDE BENDS

Somatic side bends are gentle exercises designed to stretch and release tension along the sides of the body. Here's a step-by-step guide on how to perform somatic side bends:

Somatic Side Bends Exercise:

• Comfortable Position: Stand or sit comfortably in an upright posture. Ensure your spine is comfortably straight, and your shoulders are relaxed.

• Relaxation Preparation: Allow your arms to hang naturally by your sides or rest them comfortably on your lap. Find a quiet and spacious area where you have room to move comfortably.

• Starting Position: Inhale deeply to prepare. As you exhale, gently slide one hand down the side of your body towards the knee, allowing the opposite arm to reach overhead.

• Side Bending Movement (Right Side): Inhale deeply again. As you exhale, gently bend your body to the right side, lengthening through your left side. Reach your left arm overhead and towards the right side, feeling a gentle stretch along the left side of your body.

• Stretching Sensation: Hold the stretch for a few seconds while maintaining a relaxed breath and feeling the gentle elongation along the left side of your body.

• Return to Center: Inhale deeply once more. Exhale gradually as you return to the center, releasing the stretch and allowing your body to relax.

• Side Bending Movement (Left Side): Repeat the same sequence, this time bending gently to the left side. Inhale deeply to prepare. Exhale and slide your opposite hand down the side of your body towards the knee as your other arm reaches overhead towards the left side.

• Gentle Stretch Hold: Hold the stretch for a few seconds, feeling a gentle elongation along the right side of your body while maintaining relaxed breathing.

• Return to Center and Relax: Inhale deeply again. Exhale gradually, returning your body to the center, and allow yourself to relax and settle.

Tips:

• Perform the side bends slowly and smoothly, avoiding any sudden or jerky movements.

• Focus on the quality of the stretch rather than its depth, allowing your body to stretch comfortably.

• Perform the exercise within your comfortable range of motion, without forcing the movement.

Somatic side bends can help release tension along the sides of the body and promote flexibility. Regular practice of these gentle stretches can contribute to increased relaxation and comfort in the side body area.

POSTURE, BREATHING CUE AND AWARENESS WHEN PRACTICING SOMATIC SIDE BENDS

When practicing somatic side bends, focusing on posture, syncing your breath with the movement, and maintaining awareness are essential for an effective and safe exercise. Here's an explanation of each aspect:

Posture:

• Comfortable Stance: Stand or sit comfortably in an upright and relaxed posture. Ensure your spine is comfortably straight, allowing for natural alignment without stiffness.

• Shoulder Relaxation: Keep your shoulders relaxed and away from your ears, allowing your arms to rest comfortably by your sides or on your lap.

• Natural Breathing Rhythm: Begin the side bends by taking a few deep, calming breaths to center yourself and establish a relaxed breathing pattern.

• Syncing Breath with Movement: Inhale deeply before initiating the side bend movement. Exhale gradually and steadily as you perform each side bend, allowing the exhalation to accompany the bending motion.

• Focused Attention on Stretch Sensations: Direct your attention to the sensations along the sides of your body as you perform each side bend. Notice the gentle stretching sensation along the length of the side being stretched.

• Sensory Awareness: Be mindful of any areas of tension, discomfort, or release in the side body muscles during the stretches. Observe the changes in sensation as you perform each side bend, paying attention to the quality of the stretch.

• Gentle and Controlled Movement: Perform the side bends slowly and smoothly, emphasizing a gentle and controlled range of motion. Avoid any abrupt or forceful movements, allowing the body to stretch gradually and comfortably.

• Breath and Body Connection: Use your breath as a guide to accompany the movement, ensuring a relaxed and steady breath pattern throughout the side bends. Sync your awareness of the stretching movement with the natural rhythm of your breath, promoting relaxation.

Tips:

• Maintain a relaxed and non-strained posture throughout the side bends, focusing specifically on the movement along the sides of your body.

• Adjust the depth of the side bends to your comfort level, avoiding any discomfort or strain.

• Perform the stretches at a pace that allows you to remain present and aware of the sensations along the sides of your body.

By maintaining a relaxed posture, syncing breath with movement, and fostering sensory awareness, somatic side bends can help alleviate tension and promote relaxation along the sides of the body.

STEP-BY-STEP INSTRUCTIONS FOR SOMATIC HIP CIRCLES

Somatic hip circles are gentle exercises designed to increase mobility and release tension in the hips. Here's a step-by-step guide on how to perform somatic hip circles:

Somatic Hip Circles Exercise:

• Comfortable Position: Stand with your feet comfortably apart, wider than your hips, maintaining a relaxed but stable stance.

• Relaxation Preparation: Allow your arms to hang naturally by your sides, keeping your shoulders relaxed and away from your ears.

• Starting Position: Inhale deeply to prepare. As you exhale, place your hands on your hips for stability and support.

• Hip Circles (Clockwise Direction): Inhale deeply again. As you exhale, begin to tilt your pelvis forward slightly and shift your hips to the right, initiating a circular movement. Continue the circular motion by moving your hips back, to the left, forward, and completing the circle to the starting point.

• Smooth and Controlled Movement: Perform the hip circle movement smoothly and gently, emphasizing a controlled range of motion. Keep your upper body relatively still and allow your hips to lead the movement.

• Breathing and Awareness: Maintain a relaxed and steady breath pattern throughout the hip circles. Be mindful of the sensations in your hips and the movement of your pelvis as you perform the circles.

• Hip Circles (Counterclockwise Direction): Inhale deeply once more. Exhale and reverse the movement, initiating the circle by shifting your hips to the left, then back, to the right, forward, and completing the circle to the starting position.

• Repeat the Movement: Continue to perform the hip circles in both directions, alternating between clockwise and counterclockwise circles.

Tips:

• Perform the hip circles slowly and smoothly, without forcing the movement or causing discomfort.

• Focus on the quality of the movement, allowing your hips to move comfortably through the circles.

• If you experience any discomfort or pain, reduce the range of motion or the speed of the circles.

Somatic hip circles can help increase mobility and flexibility in the hips while releasing tension in this area. Regular practice of these gentle movements can contribute to improved hip mobility and comfort.

Practicing somatic hip circles involves maintaining a relaxed posture, syncing your breath with the movement, and fostering awareness throughout the exercise. Here's an explanation of each aspect:

Posture:

• Comfortable Stance: Stand with your feet comfortably apart, wider than your hips, maintaining a relaxed but stable stance. Keep your spine comfortably straight, allowing for natural alignment without stiffness.

• Shoulder Relaxation: Keep your shoulders relaxed and away from your ears. Allow your arms to rest comfortably by your sides or place your hands on your hips for stability.

Breathing Cue:

• Natural Breathing Rhythm: Begin the hip circles by taking a few deep, calming breaths to center yourself and establish a relaxed breathing pattern.

• Syncing Breath with Movement: Inhale deeply before initiating the hip circles. Exhale gradually and steadily as you perform each circular movement of the hips, coordinating the breath with the motion.

• Focused Attention on Hip Movements: Direct your attention to the sensations in your hips and pelvis as you perform each hip circle. Notice the circular movement of your hips and the shifting of your pelvis in a smooth and controlled manner.

• Sensory Awareness: Be mindful of any areas of tension, discomfort, or release in the hip muscles during the circles. Observe the changes in sensation as you perform the hip circles, paying attention to the quality and range of motion.

• Gentle and Controlled Movement: Perform the hip circles slowly and smoothly, emphasizing a gentle and controlled range of motion. Allow your hips to move comfortably through the circles without forcing the movement.

• Breath and Body Connection: Use your breath as a guide to accompany the movement, ensuring a relaxed and steady breath pattern throughout the hip circles. Sync your awareness of the hip movement with the natural rhythm of your breath, promoting relaxation.

Tips:

• Maintain a relaxed posture throughout the hip circles, focusing specifically on the movement in your hips and pelvis.

• Adjust the speed and depth of the circles to your comfort level, avoiding any discomfort or strain.

• Perform the circles at a pace that allows you to remain present and aware of the sensations in your hips.

By maintaining a relaxed posture, syncing breath with movement, and fostering sensory awareness, somatic hip circles can help increase hip mobility and release tension in the hip muscles.

STEP-BY-STEP GUIDE TO SOMATIC KNEE-TO-CHEST STRETCH

Somatic knee-to-chest stretches are gentle exercises designed to stretch the lower back, hips, and glutes while promoting relaxation. Here's a step-by-step guide on how to perform somatic knee-to-chest stretches:

Somatic Knee-to-Chest Stretch:

• Comfortable Position: Lie down on your back on a comfortable surface, such as a yoga mat or a carpeted floor.

• Relaxation Preparation: Ensure your body is relaxed, and your arms are resting comfortably by your sides.

• Starting Position: Bend your knees, keeping your feet flat on the floor or mat. Inhale deeply to prepare for the stretch.

• Single Knee-to-Chest: Exhale gradually and gently bring one knee toward your chest, using your hands to hug the knee gently. Keep the other leg bent with the foot flat on the ground or extend it along the floor for added comfort.

• Hold the knee close to your chest with a comfortable grip, feeling a gentle stretch in the lower back and hip of the stretched leg.

• Relaxed Breathing: Maintain a relaxed breath pattern, breathing naturally and comfortably as you hold the stretch.

• Awareness and Sensations: Be mindful of the sensations in your lower back, hip, and glutes as you perform the stretch. Notice the gentle elongation and relaxation in the stretched muscles.

• Hold and Release: Hold the knee-to-chest position for about 20-30 seconds, or longer if it feels comfortable and relaxing. Gradually release the stretched leg and return it to the starting position, keeping both feet flat on the floor.

• Repeat on the Other Side: Perform the knee-to-chest stretch with the other leg, following the same steps.

Tips:

• Avoid forcing the stretch; it should be gentle and comfortable, without causing any pain.

• Perform the stretch slowly and gradually, allowing your muscles to relax into the movement.

• Adapt the stretch to your comfort level by adjusting the intensity or duration as needed.

Somatic knee-to-chest stretches can help alleviate tension in the lower back and promote relaxation in the hip and gluteal muscles. Regular practice of these gentle stretches can contribute to improved flexibility and comfort in the lower back area.

POSTURE, BREATHING CUE AND AWARENESS WHEN PRACTICING SOMATIC KNEE-TO-CHEST STRETCH

When practicing the somatic knee-to-chest stretch, it's important to focus on maintaining a relaxed posture, syncing your breath with the movement, and fostering awareness throughout the exercise. Here's an explanation of each aspect:

Posture:

• Supine Position: Lie down comfortably on your back on a yoga mat or a comfortable surface. Keep your body relaxed, with your arms resting gently by your sides.

• Leg Positioning: Bend your knees, keeping your feet flat on the floor or mat. Ensure your spine is comfortably aligned and your lower back is resting on the ground.

Breathing Cue:

• Natural Breathing Rhythm: Begin the knee-to-chest stretch by taking a few deep, calming breaths to relax and center yourself.

• Syncing Breath with Movement: Inhale deeply to prepare for the stretch. Exhale gradually as you bring one knee toward your chest, using your hands to hug the knee gently.

Awareness:

• Focused Attention on Stretch Sensations: Direct your attention to the sensations in your lower back, hip, and glutes as you perform the stretch. Notice the gentle elongation and stretching sensation in the muscles of the stretched leg.

• Sensory Awareness: Be mindful of any areas of tension, discomfort, or release in the lower back, hip, and gluteal muscles during the stretch. Observe the changes in sensation as you hold the knee-to-chest position.

• Relaxed Breathing and Muscle Relaxation: Maintain a relaxed breath pattern throughout the stretch, allowing your body to relax and sink deeper into the stretch. As you exhale, try to release any tension you might feel in the stretched muscles.

• Hold and Release: Hold the knee-to-chest position for about 20-30 seconds, or longer if comfortable, maintaining relaxed breathing. Gradually release the stretched leg, returning it to the starting position with both feet flat on the floor.

Tips:

• Perform the knee-to-chest stretch slowly and gently, without causing any discomfort or pain.

• Adapt the stretch to your comfort level, adjusting the intensity or duration as needed.

• Breathe naturally and try to relax into the stretch, allowing the muscles to release tension gradually.

By maintaining a relaxed posture, syncing breath with movement, and fostering sensory awareness, somatic knee-to-chest stretches can help alleviate tension in the lower back and promote relaxation in the hip and gluteal muscles.

STEP-BY-STEP INSTRUCTIONS FOR FULL BODY RELAXATION SCAN

A full-body relaxation scan, often used in mindfulness or meditation practices, involves systematically focusing on different parts of the body to induce a state of relaxation. Here's a step-by-step guide:

Full-Body Relaxation Scan:

Comfortable Position:

• Find a quiet and comfortable space where you can lie down or sit in a relaxed position.

• Close your eyes gently, if comfortable, or keep them softly focused on a spot.

Initial Relaxation:

• Take a few deep breaths, inhaling slowly through your nose and exhaling gently through your mouth, releasing any tension as you breathe out.

Start at the Feet:

• Focus your attention on your feet. Bring awareness to your toes, the soles, and the heels. Notice any sensations, warmth, or tingling.

• Inhale and consciously relax your feet. Exhale, letting go of any tension.

Progress Upwards:

• Gradually move your attention upward, directing it to your ankles, calves, and shins. Notice the sensations in these areas and consciously relax them.

• Inhale and as you exhale, release any tension in your lower legs.

Continue to the Knees and Thighs:

• Shift your focus to your knees and thighs. Feel the weight of your legs and any sensations present.

• Inhale deeply, and as you exhale, intentionally relax the muscles around your knees and thighs.

Move to the Pelvis and Hips:

• Bring your attention to your pelvis and hips. Notice the contact points with the surface you're resting on.

• Inhale, allowing these areas to relax with the exhale, releasing any held tension.

Focus on the Abdomen and Lower Back:

• Shift your awareness to your abdomen and lower back. Feel the rise and fall of your breath here.

• Inhale deeply, and as you exhale, consciously let go of any tightness or discomfort in this region.

Proceed to the Chest and Upper Back:

• Bring attention to your chest and upper back. Feel the expansion and contraction with each breath.

• Inhale slowly, allowing your chest to expand, and exhale, releasing any tension in the upper body.

Move Up to the Shoulders and Arms:

• Direct your focus to your shoulders, arms, and hands. Notice any sensations, warmth, or tingling in these areas.

• Inhale deeply, and as you exhale, consciously relax the muscles in your shoulders, arms, and hands.

Transition to the Neck and Head:

• Finally, concentrate on your neck, face, and head. Feel the weight of your head resting against the surface.

• Inhale and exhale, allowing the neck and facial muscles to soften and release any remaining tension.

Overall Body Awareness:

• Take a moment to shift your focus to your entire body. Notice the sense of relaxation and any areas that might still hold tension.

• Inhale deeply, and with each exhale, imagine letting go of any residual stress or discomfort.

• When ready, gently deepen your breath. Slowly wiggle your fingers and toes, and gradually transition back to a more awake state.

Tips:

• Practice this relaxation scan at your own pace, spending as much time on each body part as needed.

• Stay present and allow yourself to experience the sensations in each area without judgment.

• Practice regularly to enhance your ability to relax and release tension throughout your body.

This full-body relaxation scan can be an effective way to release tension, promote relaxation, and cultivate mindfulness throughout your entire body.

POSTURE, BREATHING CUE AND AWARENESS WHEN PRACTICING FULL BODY RELAXATION SCAN

When practicing a full-body relaxation scan, focusing on posture, syncing your breath with relaxation, and fostering awareness throughout the process are key. Here's an explanation of each aspect:

Posture:

• Comfortable Position: Find a quiet and comfortable space where you can lie down on your back or sit in a relaxed position. If lying down, ensure your body is supported and your spine is in a neutral position. If sitting, sit comfortably with your spine erect but not tense.

• Relaxed Body Alignment: Let your arms rest gently by your sides if lying down, or place your hands on your lap if sitting. Allow your legs to rest comfortably, uncrossed and relaxed.

Breathing Cue:

• Initial Breathing Awareness: Start by taking a few slow and deep breaths. Inhale deeply through your nose, feeling your abdomen rise. Exhale slowly and completely through your mouth, releasing any tension with each breath out.

• Syncing Breath with Relaxation: As you focus on each body part during the scan, sync your breath with relaxation. Inhale deeply and as you exhale, consciously release tension from that specific body area.

• Focused Attention on Body Parts: Direct your attention systematically to different parts of your body, starting from the feet and moving upward. Notice any sensations, warmth, tension, or relaxation in each body part as you focus on it.

• Mindfulness and Sensory Awareness: Be mindful of the present moment, observing the sensations in each body area without judgment or attempting to change anything. Cultivate a heightened sense of awareness, acknowledging any feelings or sensations that arise during the relaxation scan.

• Intentional Relaxation and Release: With each exhalation, intentionally relax the muscles in the specific body area you're focusing on. Let go of any tightness or tension.

• Overall Body Awareness: Toward the end of the scan, broaden your awareness to encompass your entire body. Observe the overall sensation of relaxation or any remaining areas of tension.

Tips:

• Maintain a relaxed posture throughout the relaxation scan, allowing your body to rest comfortably.

• Breathe naturally and use your breath as a guide to release tension from each body part.

• Practice the scan slowly and mindfully, spending sufficient time on each body area to encourage relaxation.

By focusing on posture, syncing breath with relaxation, and fostering awareness throughout the body, a full-body relaxation scan can effectively promote relaxation, reduce tension, and enhance overall mindfulness and body awareness.

STEP-BY-STEP GUIDE TO PROGRESSIVE MUSCLE RELAXATION

Progressive Muscle Relaxation (PMR) is a relaxation technique that involves tensing and then relaxing specific muscle groups to release physical tension. Here's a step-by-step guide to practice PMR:

Progressive Muscle Relaxation:

Comfortable Position:

• Find a quiet and comfortable place to sit or lie down. Loosen any tight clothing and remove distractions.

Breathing Awareness:

• Start with a few deep breaths, inhaling slowly through your nose and exhaling through your mouth. Allow your body to begin relaxing.

Focus on Muscle Groups:

• Begin with your toes. Curl them tightly and hold the tension for about 5-10 seconds. Feel the tension but avoid straining or causing discomfort.

• Release the tension suddenly and completely, allowing the muscles to relax completely for 20-30 seconds. Focus on the feeling of relaxation.

Progress through Muscle Groups:

• Gradually move upward, tensing and relaxing different muscle groups in your body. For example: feet and toes, calf muscles, thighs, buttocks, abdomen, hands and fingers, arms and biceps, shoulders, neck, jaw, and forehead.

• Tense each muscle group for 5-10 seconds, then release and relax for 20-30 seconds before moving to the next group.

Tension and Relaxation Technique:

• As you tense each muscle group, focus on the sensation of tension. Feel the muscles tightening but avoid any strain or pain.

• When you release the tension, let go completely. Pay attention to the contrast between tension and relaxation.

Mindful Breathing:

• Throughout the exercise, maintain slow, deep breaths. Inhale calmly during muscle tension and exhale gently during relaxation.

Complete the Cycle:

• Once you've gone through all muscle groups, take a few moments to enjoy the overall sense of relaxation throughout your body.

• If any areas still feel tense, revisit them briefly and repeat the tension-relaxation sequence.

Closure and Return:

• Gradually transition back to an awake state. Stretch gently if needed, wiggle your fingers and toes, and slowly open your eyes if they were closed.

Tips:

• Be mindful of any pain or discomfort while tensing muscles and adjust the tension level accordingly.

• Practice regularly for increased effectiveness in releasing tension.

• Keep the pace slow and controlled, focusing on each muscle group and the contrast between tension and relaxation.

Progressive Muscle Relaxation is an effective method to relieve stress and induce relaxation. With practice, it can help you become more aware of tension in your body and learn to release it consciously.

POSTURE, BREATHING CUE AND AWARENESS WHEN PRACTICING PROGRESSIVE MUSCLE RELAXATION

Practicing Progressive Muscle Relaxation (PMR) involves maintaining a comfortable posture, syncing breath with muscle tension and relaxation, and fostering awareness throughout the exercise. Here's a breakdown of each aspect:

Posture:

Comfortable Position:

• Find a quiet and comfortable place to sit or lie down. Ensure your body is well-supported, allowing for relaxation without discomfort.

• Lie down on your back with arms by your sides, palms facing up, or sit comfortably in a chair with feet flat on the floor, spine straight but not rigid.

Loosen Muscles:

• Let go of any tension in your body. Loosen tight clothing and make sure you're not holding any unnecessary tension in your muscles.

Breathing Cue:

• Deep Breathing Awareness: Start with slow, deep breaths. Inhale deeply through your nose, filling your lungs with air. Exhale slowly and completely through your mouth, releasing tension with each exhale.

• Syncing Breath with Tension and Relaxation: Inhale gently before tensing a muscle group, preparing for the tension phase. Exhale slowly and completely while consciously relaxing the muscles during the relaxation phase.

Awareness:

• Focused Attention on Muscle Groups: Concentrate on the specific muscle group you're targeting for tension and relaxation. Direct your attention to the sensations during tension and the subsequent feeling of relaxation in that muscle group.

• Tension and Release Technique: During the tensing phase, focus on the feeling of tension in the specific muscle group, but avoid causing discomfort or strain. When releasing the tension, consciously let go completely and feel the muscles relax and soften.

• Mindful Sensory Awareness: Observe and be mindful of any changes in sensation, such as the contrast between tension and relaxation in the muscle groups. Notice the difference in how the muscles feel when they are tense versus when they are relaxed.

• Breath and Body Connection: Use your breath as a guide to accompany the tension and relaxation phases, syncing it with the muscle movements. Cultivate a heightened sense of body awareness by paying attention to how your body responds to tension and relaxation.

Tips:

• Maintain a relaxed posture throughout the PMR session, allowing your body to rest comfortably.

• Breathe naturally and rhythmically, coordinating your breath with the tension and relaxation of each muscle group.

• Stay present and focused on the sensations in each muscle group, promoting relaxation and awareness throughout the exercise.

By focusing on posture, syncing breath with muscle tension and relaxation, and fostering sensory awareness, PMR can effectively help release tension and induce relaxation throughout the body.

Diaphragmatic breathing, also known as belly breathing or deep breathing, is a technique that involves breathing deeply into the belly, engaging the diaphragm muscle to promote relaxation and reduce stress. Here's a step-by-step guide:

Diaphragmatic Breathing Technique:

• Comfortable Position: Find a comfortable and quiet place to sit or lie down. You can either sit in a chair with your back straight or lie down on your back on a flat surface.

• Relaxation Preparation: Loosen any tight clothing and place one hand on your chest and the other hand on your abdomen, just below your ribcage, to feel the movement of your breath.

• Breathe Naturally: Start by taking a few normal breaths, inhaling and exhaling through your nose. Notice the natural rhythm of your breathing.

• Engage Diaphragmatic Breathing: Inhale slowly and deeply through your nose. As you breathe in, focus on expanding your abdomen instead of raising your chest. Feel your stomach rise as you inhale. Aim to fill your lower lungs by allowing the diaphragm to move downward, pushing the abdominal organs out gently.

• Exhale Slowly: Exhale slowly through your mouth or nose, whichever is more comfortable for you. Let the air out gently, feeling your abdomen fall as you breathe out. Try to make your exhalation longer than your inhalation, taking your time to release the breath fully.

• Maintain a Rhythm: Continue breathing deeply and rhythmically, allowing your breath to be smooth and relaxed. Aim for a comfortable pace, without straining or forcing the breath.

• Awareness of Breathing Pattern: Pay attention to the movement of your abdomen and the sensation of the breath entering and leaving your body. Try to make your breathing more abdominal and less chest-oriented.

• Practice Regularly: Practice diaphragmatic breathing for several minutes, gradually extending the duration as you become more comfortable with the technique. Aim for at least five minutes of diaphragmatic breathing daily to experience its benefits.

Tips:

• It might take some practice to fully engage in diaphragmatic breathing. Be patient and allow yourself time to become comfortable with the technique.

• Practice in a calm environment to maximize the relaxation benefits of deep breathing.

• You can incorporate diaphragmatic breathing into your daily routine, such as before bedtime or upon waking up, to promote relaxation and reduce stress.

By practicing diaphragmatic breathing regularly, you can effectively reduce stress, promote relaxation, and improve overall well-being by engaging in a deeper, more intentional breathing pattern.

POSTURE, BREATHING CUE AND AWARENESS WHEN PRACTICING DIAPHRAGMATIC BREATHING

Practicing diaphragmatic breathing involves focusing on posture, syncing breath with abdominal movement, and fostering awareness throughout the exercise. Here's a detailed explanation of each aspect:

Posture:

• Comfortable Position: Find a quiet and comfortable place to sit or lie down. You can sit in a chair with your back straight or lie down on your back on a flat surface. Keep your body relaxed yet aligned. Ensure your head, neck, and spine are in a neutral position.

• Relaxed Muscles: Relax your shoulders and facial muscles. Allow your hands to rest gently on your lap or by your sides, wherever you feel most comfortable.

• Natural Breathing Awareness: Start with a few natural breaths, inhaling and exhaling through your nose. Notice the regular rhythm of your breathing.

• Engaging Diaphragmatic Breathing: Inhale slowly and deeply through your nose. As you breathe in, focus on expanding your abdomen instead of raising your chest. Feel your stomach rise or expand outward as your diaphragm contracts and pushes downward, allowing air to fill your lower lungs.

• Exhale Gradually: Exhale slowly through your mouth or nose, whichever feels more comfortable for you. Allow your abdomen to fall naturally as you breathe out. Try to prolong the exhalation, allowing the breath to leave your body fully and gently.

Awareness:

• Focus on Abdominal Movement: Direct your attention to the movement of your abdomen. Notice the rise and fall with each breath. Be mindful of the expansion and contraction of your abdomen as you inhale and exhale deeply.

• Sensory Awareness of Breath: Pay attention to the sensation of the breath entering and leaving your body. Notice the flow of air in and out of your nostrils.

• Mindful Breathing Rhythm: Maintain a steady and rhythmic breathing pattern. Emphasize a smooth transition between inhalation and exhalation.

Tips:

• Relaxation is key. Avoid any tension or stiffness in your body, especially in your shoulders and chest.

• Practice diaphragmatic breathing regularly, allowing yourself to become more comfortable with the technique over time.

• You can practice diaphragmatic breathing for a few minutes several times a day to promote relaxation and reduce stress.

By focusing on posture, syncing breath with abdominal movement, and fostering sensory awareness, diaphragmatic breathing can effectively promote relaxation, reduce stress, and improve overall well-being through intentional, deep breathing.

STEP-BY-STEP GUIDE TO GUIDED VISUALIZATION MEDITATION

Guided visualization meditation is a practice that involves imagining peaceful scenes or scenarios, often guided by a narrator or recorded audio. It's aimed at promoting relaxation, reducing stress, and fostering a sense of calm. Here's a step-by-step guide:

Guided Visualization Meditation:

• Prepare a Quiet Space: Find a quiet and comfortable space where you won't be disturbed. Dim the lights or play calming music if it helps create a relaxing atmosphere.

• Choose a Guided Visualization: Select a guided visualization audio, meditation app, or a script that resonates with you. You can focus on nature scenes, peaceful journeys, or any visualization that promotes relaxation.

• Comfortable Position: Sit or lie down in a comfortable position. You might prefer lying on your back or sitting in a supportive chair with your feet flat on the ground and your hands resting comfortably.

• Relaxation Preparation: Close your eyes gently and take a few deep breaths to center yourself and relax your body. Inhale deeply through your nose and exhale slowly through your mouth.

• Start the Guided Visualization: Follow the instructions provided by the narrator or the recorded audio. They will typically guide you through a journey or scenario, describing various calming scenes or experiences.

• Engage Your Senses: As the visualization unfolds, imagine vividly and engage your senses. Visualize colors, textures, sounds, scents, and even emotions associated with the guided scenario.

• Mindfulness and Relaxation: Remain present and immersed in the visualization. Let go of any distracting thoughts, focusing solely on the images and sensations described in the guidance.

• Deep Relaxation and Calmness: Allow the visualization to lead you to a state of deep relaxation and tranquility. Embrace the sense of peace and calmness as the visualization progresses.

• Closure and Return: Towards the end of the guided meditation, the narrator will gently guide you back to the present moment. Take a few deep breaths and slowly open your eyes.

Tips:

• Find a guided visualization that resonates with you or creates a calming experience.

• Be patient and allow yourself to immerse deeply in the visualization without judgment or pressure.

• Practice guided visualization regularly to enhance its relaxation benefits and promote a sense of inner peace.

Guided visualization meditation is a powerful tool to unwind, de-stress, and cultivate a sense of inner peace. By following the guidance and allowing yourself to immerse in the imagery, you can experience profound relaxation and mental rejuvenation.

POSTURE, BREATHING CUE AND AWARENESS WHEN PRACTICING GUIDED VISUALIZATION MEDITATION

Practicing guided visualization meditation involves focusing on posture, syncing breath with relaxation, and fostering awareness of the guided imagery. Here's a detailed explanation of each aspect:

Posture:

• Comfortable Position: Find a quiet and comfortable space where you won't be disturbed. You can sit on a cushion, chair, or lie down on a yoga mat or bed. Keep your spine comfortably straight, allowing for natural alignment without stiffness.

• Relax Your Body: Let go of any tension in your body. Allow your shoulders to relax, and place your hands comfortably on your lap or by your sides.

Breathing Cue:

• Initial Relaxation Breathing: Begin with a few deep breaths to relax your body and mind. Inhale slowly through your nose and exhale gently through your mouth, releasing any tension.

• Syncing Breath with Visualization: As the guided visualization starts, maintain a relaxed breathing pattern. Breathe naturally and rhythmically, syncing your breath with the guidance.

Awareness:

• Focused Attention on Guidance: Concentrate on the narrator's voice or the guided imagery presented to you. Let go of distractions and immerse yourself in the scenes described.

• Engage Your Senses: Visualize the scenes described vividly. Engage your imagination and try to visualize colors, textures, sounds, scents, and emotions associated with the guided scenario.

• Mindful Presence: Stay present in the moment. Be aware of the imagery as it unfolds, allowing yourself to experience each detail without judgment or attachment.

• Relaxation Response: Allow the guided visualization to lead you to a state of relaxation and calmness. Embrace the feelings of peace and tranquility conveyed by the imagery.

• Release and Return: Toward the end of the session, gradually bring your focus back to the present moment. Take a few deep breaths and gently open your eyes.

Tips:

• Maintain a relaxed posture throughout the guided visualization session, allowing your body to rest comfortably.

• Follow the guidance provided and let your imagination flow freely without any pressure or expectations.

• Practice guided visualization regularly to improve relaxation and inner peace.

By focusing on posture, syncing breath with relaxation, and fostering awareness of the guided imagery, you can deepen your experience and gain more profound relaxation and mental rejuvenation through guided visualization meditation.

Body swaying or rocking is a relaxation technique that involves gentle rhythmic movements to promote relaxation and calmness. Here's a step-by-step guide to practicing body swaying or rocking:

Body Swaying/Rocking Technique:

• Find a Comfortable Space: Choose a quiet and safe area where you can move freely without any obstacles.

• Stand or Sit Comfortably: Stand with your feet shoulder-width apart or sit comfortably on a chair with your feet flat on the floor. Ensure your posture is relaxed and aligned.

• Relax Your Body: Relax your shoulders and let your arms hang naturally by your sides. Keep your spine comfortably straight but not rigid.

• Begin Gentle Movements: Start swaying gently from side to side or back and forth, allowing your body to move with a slow and rhythmic motion. You can allow your arms to move freely or keep them relaxed by your sides as you sway.

• Sync with Your Breath: Coordinate your movements with your breath. Inhale deeply as you sway in one direction and exhale as you sway in the opposite direction. Let the rhythm of your breath guide the rhythm of your swaying.

- Focus on Relaxation: As you sway, focus on the sensation of movement and relaxation. Feel the gentle shift in weight from one foot to the other or the movement in your torso.

- Mindful Awareness: Be present and mindful of the swaying motion. Notice how your body responds to the rhythmic movement. Allow yourself to relax further with each sway, letting go of any tension or stress.

- Maintain a Comfortable Pace: Continue swaying or rocking at a pace that feels comfortable for you. Let the movement be soothing and calming.

- Gradually Slow Down: After a few minutes, gradually slow down the swaying motion. Allow yourself to come to a gentle stop.

- Closure and Relaxation: Take a moment to stand or sit quietly, noticing any sensations or feelings of relaxation in your body. Take a few deep breaths and acknowledge the calming effect of the body swaying.

Tips:

- Practice body swaying in a way that feels natural and comfortable for your body.

- Experiment with different directions (side-to-side, front-to-back) and find the rhythm that works best for you.

• Incorporate body swaying into your relaxation routine or use it as a brief break during stressful moments to calm your mind and body.

Body swaying or rocking can be a simple yet effective technique to induce relaxation and ease tension in the body. The gentle rhythmic movement can help calm the mind and promote a sense of tranquility.

POSTURE, BREATHING CUE AND AWARENESS WHEN PRACTICING BODY SWAYING OR ROCKING

When practicing body swaying or rocking for relaxation, it's essential to focus on posture, sync your breath with the movement, and maintain mindful awareness. Here's a detailed explanation of each aspect:

Posture:

• Comfortable Position: Stand with your feet hip-width apart or sit comfortably on a chair with your feet flat on the floor. Keep your spine comfortably straight but not rigid, allowing for a relaxed and aligned posture.

• Relaxed Body Alignment: Relax your shoulders and arms. Let your arms hang naturally by your sides if standing, or rest them comfortably on your lap if sitting. Keep your neck and head in a comfortable and neutral position.

• Initiate Relaxation Breathing: Begin with a few deep breaths to relax your body. Inhale slowly through your nose and exhale gently through your mouth, releasing tension with each exhale.

• Syncing Breath with Movement: Coordinate your swaying or rocking movements with your breath. Inhale deeply as you sway in one direction, and exhale as you sway in the opposite direction. Let the rhythm of your breath guide the rhythm of your swaying.

Awareness:

• Focus on Rhythmic Movement: Concentrate on the gentle and rhythmic swaying or rocking motion. Allow your body to move naturally and fluidly with the rhythm you've established.

• Mindful Sensory Awareness: Be present in the moment, paying attention to the sensation of movement. Notice how your body responds to the swaying motion. Feel the subtle shifts in weight as you sway from one side to another or the gentle movement throughout your body.

• Relaxation Response: Embrace the soothing and calming effect of the movement. Allow yourself to relax further with each sway, letting go of any tension or stress.

• Focused Attention: Direct your focus to the present experience of swaying. Let go of distractions and immerse yourself fully in the rhythm and sensation of the movement.

Tips:

• Keep your movements gentle and relaxed, allowing your body to sway naturally.

• Breathe deeply and rhythmically, syncing your breath with the swaying motion for a more calming effect.

• Practice body swaying or rocking regularly as part of your relaxation routine to experience its benefits fully.

By focusing on posture, syncing breath with movement, and maintaining mindful awareness, body swaying or rocking can effectively induce relaxation, ease tension, and promote a sense of calmness and tranquility.

CHAPTER FOUR

HOW BEGINNERS CAN PROGRESS IN THEIR SOMATIC PRACTICE

For beginners in somatic practice, progression involves gradually deepening one's understanding and experience with somatic exercises while integrating them into daily life. Here are some steps beginners can follow to progress in their somatic practice:

1. Consistency and Patience:

• Start Small: Begin with short sessions, maybe 10-15 minutes, and gradually increase the duration as you become more comfortable.

• Regular Practice: Aim for consistency in your practice. Even a few minutes of somatic exercises every day can yield benefits.

2. Body Awareness and Mindfulness:

• Focused Attention: Pay close attention to the sensations in your body during exercises. Heighten your awareness of how each movement feels.

• Mindfulness Practice: Incorporate mindfulness techniques into your routine to complement somatic exercises and deepen body awareness.

3. Gentle Progression in Exercises:

• Beginner-friendly Exercises: Start with simple and gentle exercises that focus on body awareness and relaxation.

• Gradual Complexity: As you become more familiar, slowly introduce more complex movements or sequences. Allow yourself to adapt and progress naturally.

4. Integration into Daily Life:

• Mindful Movement: Apply somatic principles to everyday activities. Pay attention to how you move, sit, stand, or perform daily tasks.

• Mind-Body Connection: Practice integrating body awareness into routine activities, enhancing your overall mindfulness.

5. Seeking Guidance and Learning:

• Explore Resources: Utilize books, online resources, videos, or consider attending classes or workshops led by somatic practitioners.

• Expert Guidance: If possible, seek guidance from a qualified somatic practitioner or instructor to deepen your understanding and practice.

6. Listening to Your Body:

• Respect Your Limits: Be mindful of your body's limits and avoid pushing yourself into discomfort or pain.

• Modify as Needed: Modify exercises if required to suit your comfort level and physical capabilities.

7. Reflect and Adapt:

• Self-Reflection: Take time to reflect on how somatic practice affects you. Notice any changes in your body awareness, stress levels, or overall well-being.

• Adaptation: Adjust your practice based on your experiences. Be open to trying new exercises or approaches that resonate with you.

8. Long-Term Commitment:

• Long-Term Approach: Embrace somatic practice as a journey rather than a destination. Understand that progress takes time and commitment.

• Celebrate Milestones: Acknowledge and celebrate your progress, whether it's improved body awareness, reduced tension, or enhanced relaxation.

By embracing a gradual and consistent approach, listening to your body, seeking guidance when needed, and integrating somatic principles into your daily life, beginners can progressively deepen their somatic practice and experience its benefits more profoundly over time.

Gradually introducing more complex exercises in somatic practice requires a mindful and progressive approach. Here's a step-by-step guide to help beginners integrate these more intricate movements:

1. Foundational Exercises Mastery:

• Establish a Base: Begin with foundational exercises like body scans, gentle stretches, or basic breathing techniques.

• Consistency: Practice these foundational exercises regularly to build body awareness and familiarity with somatic principles.

2. Incremental Progression:

• Small Modifications: Start by making slight modifications or variations to familiar exercises. For instance, extend the duration, range of motion, or add a gentle twist to a basic stretch.

• Gradual Complexity: Introduce slight alterations, focusing on engaging different muscle groups or exploring variations in body positioning.

3. Controlled Breathing Integration:

• Breath Coordination: Incorporate controlled breathing techniques into movements. For instance, sync specific movements with inhalation or exhalation to deepen the mind-body connection.

• Breath Manipulation: Experiment with varying the pace or depth of breathing while performing more intricate movements.

4. Sequencing and Combinations:

• Sequence Building: Combine multiple exercises or movements into a sequence. Start with simple combinations and progress to more elaborate sequences.

• Flow Creation: Aim for fluidity in transitions between movements, ensuring a seamless flow while maintaining mindfulness.

5. Incorporating Balance and Stability:

• Focus on Balance: Introduce exercises that challenge balance or stability slightly. This might involve standing on one leg while performing a somatic movement or integrating gentle weight shifts.

• Mindful Stability: Emphasize body awareness and stability while attempting these exercises, ensuring safety and gradual improvement.

6. Mindful Exploration:

• Expanded Exploration: Expand your exploration to different body parts or movements. Experiment with more complex exercises that engage larger muscle groups or intricate joint movements.

• Mindful Experimentation: Approach these new exercises mindfully, paying close attention to sensations and responses within your body.

7. Incorporating Guided Sessions or Expert Guidance:

• Guided Instruction: Utilize resources like guided sessions or classes tailored for progressive learning.

• Expert Guidance: Seek guidance from a somatic practitioner or instructor to ensure proper technique and safe progression.

Tips:

• Mindful Progress: Approach complex exercises with mindfulness, maintaining focus on bodily sensations and alignment.

• Listen to Your Body: Respect your body's limits and avoid pushing beyond your comfort level or experiencing pain.

• Gradual Integration: Introduce complexity at a pace that feels comfortable and allows for adaptation over time.

By gradually incorporating more complex exercises with mindfulness, patience, and a progressive mindset, beginners can expand their somatic practice, fostering enhanced body awareness, flexibility, and relaxation.

MORE COMPLEX SOMATIC EXERCISES FOR BEGINNERS

Here are some more complex somatic exercises that beginners can gradually integrate into their practice. Remember to approach these exercises mindfully, respecting your body's limits, and gradually increasing intensity or complexity as you become more comfortable:

1. Somatic Leg Lifts:

• Exercise: Lie on your back with legs extended. Lift one leg slowly, keeping it straight without locking the knee. Lower it back down with control.

• Focus: Engage core muscles, feel the movement from hip to toe, and maintain relaxation in the rest of your body.

2. Somatic Cat-Cow Stretch:

• Exercise: Start on hands and knees. Arch your back upwards (Cat Pose) while tucking your chin. Then, lower your belly down, lifting your head and tailbone (Cow Pose).

• Focus: Coordinate movement with breath - inhale in Cat Pose, exhale in Cow Pose. Focus on the spinal stretch and breath synchronization.

3. Somatic Forward Fold:

• Exercise: Stand with feet hip-width apart. Slowly bend forward from the hips, letting your upper body hang. Keep knees slightly bent. Relax neck and shoulders.

• Focus: Feel the release in the lower back and hamstrings. Use breath to deepen the stretch, exhaling as you fold forward.

4. Somatic Hip Opener:

• Exercise: Sit on the floor with legs extended. Bend one knee and cross the foot over the opposite thigh. Gently press the crossed knee away from the body.

• Focus: Feel the stretch in the hips and buttocks. Maintain relaxation in the upper body and breathe deeply into the stretch.

5. Somatic Seated Twist:

• Exercise: Sit cross-legged or on a chair. Inhale, lengthen your spine, exhale, twist your torso to one side, placing the opposite hand on the outer thigh.

• Focus: Feel the twist starting from the base of the spine. Inhale to lengthen, exhale to twist deeper, maintaining relaxation in the neck and shoulders.

6. Somatic Shoulder Stand:

• Exercise: Lie on your back, lift legs, and lower back off the ground, supporting your lower back with your hands. Extend legs upward, aligning them with your torso.

• Focus: Engage core muscles for stability. Feel the inversion and breathe deeply while relaxing the neck and shoulders.

7. Somatic Bridge Pose:

• Exercise: Lie on your back, bend knees, feet hip-width apart. Inhale, lift hips towards the ceiling, pressing feet into the floor. Hold briefly, then lower hips.

• Focus: Feel the stretch in the chest, hips, and thighs. Focus on the upward movement while maintaining relaxation in the upper body.

Tips:

• Start with caution and gradually increase the intensity or duration of these exercises.

• Focus on relaxation and mindful movement, ensuring you're not straining or forcing any positions.

• Use breath awareness to deepen the stretches and movements, syncing breath with motion when appropriate.

These exercises can offer a deeper exploration of movement and body awareness. Always listen to your body and modify or pause if you experience discomfort. Seek guidance from a certified somatic practitioner if needed to ensure proper technique and safety.

STEP-BY-STEP GUIDE OF SOMATIC LEG LIFTS

Somatic leg lifts are a beneficial exercise for improving body awareness, engaging core muscles, and strengthening the legs. Here's a step-by-step guide to performing somatic leg lifts:

Somatic Leg Lifts:

• Initial Position: Lie on your back on a comfortable surface, such as a yoga mat or a carpeted floor. Extend your legs comfortably along the floor. Rest your arms by your sides with palms facing down for support.

• Body Awareness and Relaxation: Take a moment to relax your entire body. Close your eyes if comfortable, and focus on releasing tension from your muscles.

• Engage Core Muscles: Bring your attention to your core muscles – the abdominal area and lower back. Engage these muscles slightly to support your lower back.

• Starting the Leg Lift: Inhale deeply and slowly lift one leg off the floor, keeping it straight but not locked at the knee. Lift it to a comfortable height while maintaining control. Use your core muscles to assist in the movement, focusing on the engagement rather than the height of the lift.

• Mindful Movement: Exhale slowly as you lower the lifted leg back to the floor, maintaining control throughout the descent. Feel the movement of the leg as it lowers, noticing the engagement in your core and the sensation in the leg muscles.

• Switching Sides: Repeat the same movement with the opposite leg. Inhale as you lift the leg, and exhale as you lower it back down.

• Body Awareness and Relaxation: Take a moment to rest and relax your body, allowing the effects of the leg lifts to settle in. Focus on any sensations in your legs and the engagement of your core muscles.

• Repetition and Sets: Perform several repetitions of leg lifts on each side, starting with a manageable number and gradually increasing as you become more comfortable. Aim for a balanced number of lifts on both legs.

Tips:

• Focus on the engagement of core muscles throughout the movement, ensuring they assist in the lift and control during the descent.

• Keep the movement slow and controlled, emphasizing quality over quantity.

• Avoid arching your lower back excessively; maintain a neutral spine position to protect your lower back.

Remember to listen to your body and perform the exercise within your comfort level. Over time, as you become more familiar with somatic leg lifts, you can gradually increase the number of repetitions or explore variations under the guidance of a certified somatic practitioner.

STEP-BY-STEP GUIDE OF SOMATIC CAT-COW STRETCH

The somatic cat-cow stretch is a wonderful exercise to mobilize the spine, enhance flexibility, and promote body awareness. Here's a step-by-step guide to performing the somatic cat-cow stretch:

Somatic Cat-Cow Stretch:

• Initial Position: Begin on your hands and knees in a tabletop position, ensuring your wrists are aligned under your shoulders and knees under your hips. Spread your fingers comfortably, with the middle fingers pointing forward.

• Body Awareness and Relaxation: Take a moment to relax your body. Close your eyes if comfortable, and focus on releasing tension from your muscles, especially in your neck and shoulders.

• Engage Core Muscles: Engage your core slightly by gently drawing your navel toward your spine. This engagement supports your lower back during the movement.

• Cow Pose (Somatic Arch): Inhale deeply as you begin the movement. Drop your belly towards the floor, lift your chest and tailbone upward, arching your back.

• Lift your head, look forward, and gently tilt your pelvis forward. Allow your stomach to move toward the floor without sinking into your shoulders.

• Mindful Movement: Exhale slowly and initiate the Cat Pose. Round your spine upward toward the ceiling, tuck your chin toward your chest, and release your head gently.

• Tilt your pelvis backward, drawing your navel toward your spine. Feel the stretch along your back as you round your spine.

• Breath Coordination: Coordinate your breath with the movement. Inhale as you transition into the Cow Pose (arch), and exhale as you move into the Cat Pose (rounding).

• Smooth Transitions: Focus on the fluidity of the movement, maintaining a slow and controlled pace as you transition between the two poses.

• Move slowly to explore the full range of motion and deepen the stretch while maintaining relaxation in the neck and shoulders.

• Repetition and Flow: Repeat the Cat-Cow stretch for several rounds, allowing your breath to guide the movement. Aim for a smooth flow between the two poses.

Tips:

• Emphasize the fluidity and mindfulness of the movement rather than focusing solely on the depth of the stretch.

• Engage your core muscles to support your spine throughout the movement, enhancing stability and control.

• Practice at your own pace, gradually increasing the number of repetitions or exploring variations as you become more comfortable.

The somatic cat-cow stretch is a gentle and effective way to mobilize the spine and increase body awareness. Listen to your body, breathe deeply, and enjoy the movement, allowing it to release tension and promote relaxation.

The somatic forward fold is an excellent exercise for gently stretching the posterior chain of the body, including the hamstrings, lower back, and shoulders. Here's a step-by-step guide:

Somatic Forward Fold:

• Initial Position: Start in a standing position with your feet about hip-width apart. Ensure a slight bend in your knees to prevent excessive strain.

• Body Awareness and Relaxation: Take a moment to relax your body. Stand tall, shoulders relaxed, and breathe deeply to release any tension.

• Engage Core Muscles: Engage your core slightly by gently drawing your navel toward your spine. This engagement helps support your lower back during the forward fold.

• Inhale for Lengthening: Inhale deeply, lengthening your spine upward, and allow your chest to open. Feel the extension from your tailbone to the crown of your head.

• Forward Folding Movement: Exhale slowly as you hinge forward at the hips, leading with your chest. Keep your back flat and extend forward rather than down, aiming to bring your chest parallel to the floor.

• Hands Placement: Let your arms hang or reach towards the floor, allowing them to relax. You can touch the floor or let your hands hang near your feet or shins, depending on your flexibility.

• Mindful Relaxation: Release any tension in your neck and shoulders. Let your head hang naturally, and relax your facial muscles.

• Breath Awareness: Breathe deeply and smoothly while holding the stretch. Inhale to maintain length in your spine, and exhale to relax into the stretch.

• Gentle Release: To come out of the stretch, engage your core muscles gently, and inhale as you slowly rise back up to a standing position.

• Body Awareness: Notice the sensations in your hamstrings, lower back, and shoulders as you return to the standing position.

Tips:

• Focus on lengthening the spine and reaching forward rather than pushing forcefully into the stretch.

• Keep a micro-bend in your knees if you feel any discomfort or strain in your hamstrings.

• Avoid forcing your body into the stretch; instead, let gravity and relaxation guide you into the forward fold.

Perform the somatic forward fold mindfully, breathing deeply, and embracing the stretch without overexertion. Gradually deepen the stretch over time as your flexibility increases, always respecting your body's limits.

STEP-BY-STEP GUIDE OF SOMATIC HIP OPENER

The somatic hip opener exercise helps improve flexibility and mobility in the hips. Here's a step-by-step guide:

Somatic Hip Opener:

• Initial Position: Start by sitting comfortably on the floor or a mat with your legs extended in front of you.

• Relaxation and Body Awareness: Take a moment to relax your body. Sit tall, allowing your spine to lengthen, and breathe deeply to release any tension.

• Engage Core Muscles: Engage your core slightly by gently drawing your navel toward your spine. This engagement helps maintain stability and support your lower back.

• Bend One Knee: Bend your right knee and cross the foot over your left thigh, placing it on the floor beside the opposite knee.

• Setting Up the Posture: Keep your spine tall and your sitting bones grounded. Adjust your position to find comfort while maintaining proper alignment.

• Gentle Pressing Movement: Press your right knee gently away from your body using your hand or elbow. Apply light pressure to feel a gentle stretch in the outer hip and thigh.

• Mindful Relaxation and Breathing: Relax your shoulders and facial muscles. Take slow, deep breaths, inhaling to create space in the hips and exhaling to relax into the stretch.

• Stay Mindful and Relax: Focus on relaxing into the stretch without forcing or bouncing. Feel the sensations in the hip area and allow the stretch to deepen gradually with each exhale.

• Switching Sides: Release the stretch slowly and return to the initial position with both legs extended. Repeat the same sequence on the opposite side by bending the left knee and crossing the foot over the right thigh.

Tips:

• Maintain an upright and relaxed posture throughout the stretch, avoiding any rounding or slumping of the back.

• Adjust the intensity of the stretch by applying more or less pressure, depending on your comfort level.

• Avoid any sharp or painful sensations. The stretch should feel like a gentle pull or opening in the outer hip area.

Remember to perform the somatic hip opener gently, respecting your body's limitations, and gradually increasing the stretch over time as your flexibility improves. Consistency in practice can help improve hip mobility and reduce tension in the hip area.

STEP-BY-STEP GUIDE OF SOMATIC SEATED TWIST

The somatic seated twist is an exercise that helps in increasing spinal mobility and promoting flexibility in the torso. Here's a step-by-step guide:

Somatic Seated Twist:

• Initial Position: Sit on the floor or on a chair with both legs extended in front of you. Keep your spine tall, shoulders relaxed, and feet grounded.

• Relaxation and Body Awareness: Take a moment to relax your body. Sit tall, allowing your spine to lengthen, and breathe deeply to release any tension.

• Bend One Knee: Bend your right knee and cross it over your left leg, placing the foot flat on the floor beside the outer thigh of your extended leg.

• Setting Up the Posture: Plant your right hand on the floor or the backrest of the chair behind you for support. Inhale and lengthen your spine upward, ensuring an erect posture.

• Twisting Movement: Exhale as you gently twist your torso to the right, using your left hand to hug the outside of your right knee. Place your right hand on the floor or the backrest of the chair, providing support and aiding the twist.

• Mindful Relaxation and Breathing: Relax your shoulders and facial muscles. Take slow, deep breaths, inhaling to lengthen the spine and exhaling to twist a bit deeper.

• Gentle Twisting Motion: Feel the stretch along the spine and the opening in the chest and shoulders. Allow the twist to deepen gradually with each exhalation.

• Maintain the Twist and Breathing: Hold the twist for a few breaths, continuing to breathe deeply and maintaining relaxation throughout your body.

• Return to Center and Switch Sides: Inhale to slowly release the twist, returning to face forward. Extend both legs and repeat the same sequence on the opposite side by crossing the left leg over the right and twisting to the left.

Tips:

• Keep your spine long and avoid collapsing or slouching during the twist.

• Use your breath to deepen the stretch, inhaling to lengthen the spine and exhaling to ease into the twist.

• Avoid any excessive or forced twisting; let the movement be gentle and within your comfort level.

Perform the somatic seated twist mindfully, focusing on the stretch along the spine and torso. Gradually deepen the twist over time as your flexibility increases, and always honor your body's limitations. Regular practice can help enhance spinal mobility and alleviate tension in the back and shoulders.

STEP-BY-STEP GUIDE OF SOMATIC SHOULDER STAND

The shoulder stand, while a yoga pose, can offer numerous benefits for the body including improved circulation, strengthening of the shoulders and core, and calming the mind. However, it's crucial to approach this pose mindfully and ensure it's suitable for your body. Here's a step-by-step guide:

Somatic Shoulder Stand:

Note: This pose may not be suitable for everyone, especially those with neck or back issues, high blood pressure, or certain medical conditions. If unsure, consult a healthcare professional or a certified yoga instructor before attempting.

• Initial Position: Begin by lying on your back on a soft surface, like a yoga mat. Keep your arms alongside your body, palms facing down.

• Body Awareness and Relaxation: Take a few moments to relax your body. Breathe deeply and allow your entire body to soften and release tension.

• Engage Core Muscles: Gently engage your core muscles by drawing your navel towards your spine. This activation supports your lower back during the pose.

• Lifting Into Shoulder Stand: Inhale deeply and, using your core strength, lift your legs towards the ceiling. Support your lower back with your hands, placing your palms against your lower back or hips for stability.

• Raising Legs Upward: Continue lifting your legs, allowing them to rise upward, aiming to bring them in line with your torso. Keep your neck and head relaxed on the floor.

• Support and Alignment: Use your hands to support your lower back and hips. Ensure your elbows are placed firmly on the ground, providing additional support.

• Mindful Breathing and Relaxation: Breathe deeply and evenly while in the pose. Allow your body to relax into the stretch, focusing on the sensations in your shoulders, core, and legs.

• Maintain the Pose: Hold the shoulder stand for a comfortable duration, being mindful of any strain or discomfort. The duration may vary based on your comfort level.

• Gentle Release: To exit the pose, slowly lower your legs back down towards the floor, one at a time, while maintaining control. Once your legs are down, rest for a moment in Savasana (corpse pose) to allow your body to readjust.

Tips:

• Avoid any jerky movements or excessive strain on the neck or shoulders.

• If uncomfortable, come out of the pose immediately and return to a neutral position.

• It's essential to learn this pose under the guidance of a certified yoga instructor to ensure proper alignment and minimize the risk of injury.

Please practice caution and ensure you're physically ready for this pose. If you have any concerns or medical conditions, it's advisable to consult with a healthcare professional before attempting the shoulder stand.

STEP-BY-STEP GUIDE OF SOMATIC BRIDGE POSE

The Bridge Pose (Setu Bandhasana) in yoga offers various benefits, including stretching the chest, neck, spine, and thighs while strengthening the back, glutes, and hamstrings. Here's a step-by-step guide to performing the Bridge Pose with a somatic approach:

Somatic Bridge Pose:

• Initial Position: Lie down on your back on a comfortable surface, such as a yoga mat, with knees bent and feet flat on the floor hip-width apart. Rest your arms alongside your body with palms facing down.

• Body Awareness and Relaxation: Take a moment to relax your body. Breathe deeply and allow your entire body to soften, releasing tension.

• Engage Core Muscles: Gently engage your core by slightly drawing your navel towards your spine. This engagement supports your lower back during the pose.

• Lifting Into the Bridge: Inhale deeply, pressing your feet firmly into the floor. Slowly lift your hips upward while maintaining contact between your feet and the ground. Lift your hips as high as comfortable, allowing your spine to arch gently.

• Support and Alignment: You can choose to interlace your fingers underneath your body, creating support for your lifted hips. Alternatively, keep your palms flat on the floor for stability.

• Mindful Breathing and Relaxation: Breathe deeply and evenly while in the pose. Allow your body to relax into the stretch, focusing on the sensations in your chest, hips, and thighs.

• Maintain the Pose: Hold the Bridge Pose for a comfortable duration, allowing your body to adapt to the stretch. Avoid overexertion or strain.

• Gentle Release: To release the pose, exhale slowly and lower your hips down to the floor with control, one vertebra at a time. Rest for a moment in a neutral position, allowing your body to readjust and relax.

Tips:

• Focus on lifting your hips using your leg muscles while keeping your shoulders and neck relaxed.

• Avoid overarching your neck or straining your back. Keep the movement smooth and controlled.

• If you experience discomfort or strain, lower your hips immediately and return to a resting position.

Perform the somatic Bridge Pose mindfully, respecting your body's limits, and gradually increasing the stretch as your body becomes more accustomed to the posture. This exercise can help enhance flexibility in the spine and hips while strengthening the posterior chain muscles.

MODIFICATIONS FOR INDIVIDUALS WITH DIFFERENT BODY TYPES, ABILITIES, OR LIMITATIONS.

Modifying yoga poses like the Bridge Pose can make them accessible and comfortable for individuals with varying body types, abilities, or limitations. Here are some modifications:

1. Use Props:

• Support Under Hips: Place a yoga block, folded blanket, or bolster under the sacrum for additional support if lifting the hips is challenging.

• Support for Head/Neck: Use a folded towel or cushion under your neck if you need extra support for the head or have neck sensitivity.

2. Partial Bridge:

• Low Bridge: If lifting the hips high is uncomfortable, lift the hips to a smaller, more manageable height. The focus is on maintaining alignment and feeling a stretch without strain.

• One-Legged Bridge: Lift one leg up towards the ceiling while maintaining the other foot on the floor to reduce intensity.

3. Hand Placement:

• Palms Down: Keep palms flat on the floor for support and stability.

• Fingers Interlaced: Interlace fingers under the body to create a supportive base for the lifted hips. Adjust hand position based on comfort.

4. Leg Positioning:

• Wider Stance: Widen the distance between your feet for more stability and balance, especially if you have a broader body structure.

• Feet Position: Experiment with different foot placements (closer or farther from the body) to find a comfortable position for lifting the hips.

5. Chair Variation:

• Supported Bridge with Chair: Sit with your back against a sturdy chair, knees bent, and feet flat on the floor. Slowly lift your hips off the ground by pushing against the chair's seat.

6. Breathing and Relaxation:

• Focus on Breathing: Place more emphasis on mindful breathing and relaxation during the pose, ensuring comfort and ease while maintaining a steady breath pattern.

• Shorter Hold: If necessary, reduce the duration of the hold in the pose, gradually increasing it as you become more comfortable.

7. Consultation:

• Seek Guidance: If you have specific physical limitations or medical conditions, consult with a healthcare professional or a certified yoga instructor for personalized modifications.

Modifications should be tailored to individual needs. It's crucial to listen to your body and adjust the pose accordingly. Yoga is about adapting the practice to suit your body rather than forcing your body into a specific shape. By exploring these modifications, individuals can experience the benefits of the Bridge Pose while honoring their unique bodies and capabilities.

COMMON MISTAKES OR CHALLENGES BEGINNERS MIGHT FACE

Beginners in yoga, particularly when attempting poses like the Bridge Pose, may encounter some common challenges or make mistakes. Here are a few:

1. Overarching the Neck:

• Mistake: Lifting the head excessively during the Bridge Pose, leading to strain or discomfort in the neck.

• Tip: Keep the neck relaxed and avoid straining by maintaining a natural alignment; avoid tilting the head too far back.

2. Overarching the Lower Back:

• Mistake: Creating an excessive arch in the lower back, which might strain the lower spine.

• Tip: Engage the core muscles slightly to support the lower back and lift the hips without overly arching the spine. Focus on a moderate lift, maintaining the natural curve of the spine.

3. Lack of Proper Support:

• Mistake: Failing to provide adequate support for the back and hips, leading to discomfort or instability during the pose.

• Tip: Use props like yoga blocks or bolsters under the sacrum or support the neck with a cushion if needed. Ensure a stable and comfortable base for the pose.

4. Shoulder Tension:

• Mistake: Holding tension in the shoulders or shrugging them up towards the ears during the pose.

• Tip: Relax the shoulders away from the ears and distribute weight evenly through the arms, maintaining a relaxed upper body.

5. Forcing the Pose:

• Mistake: Striving to achieve the highest lift without considering comfort or alignment.

• Tip: Focus on proper alignment, listen to your body, and only lift to a comfortable height without straining. Gradually work towards higher lifts as your flexibility increases.

6. Hip Instability:

• Mistake: Inadequate engagement of the core and leg muscles, leading to unstable hips during the pose.

• Tip: Engage the muscles of the legs and core to support the lift. Ensure stability by pressing firmly into the feet and engaging the glutes and hamstrings.

7. Holding the Breath:

• Mistake: Holding the breath or breathing shallowly while in the pose, leading to tension or discomfort.

• Tip: Maintain steady and relaxed breathing throughout the pose. Inhale and exhale deeply to enhance relaxation and release tension.

8. Pushing Beyond Limits:

• Mistake: Ignoring the body's signals and pushing too hard into the pose, risking strain or injury.

• Tip: Respect your body's limits. If you experience pain or discomfort, gently release from the pose or modify it to suit your comfort level.

9. Lack of Relaxation:

• Mistake: Failing to relax into the pose, which may hinder the intended benefits and cause unnecessary tension.

• Tip: Emphasize relaxation by breathing deeply and allowing the body to soften into the pose, finding a balance between effort and ease.

By being mindful of these potential challenges and mistakes, beginners can approach the Bridge Pose with greater awareness, focusing on alignment, breath, and comfort to maximize the benefits while minimizing the risk of injury or discomfort. Regular practice with attention to these aspects can enhance the experience and effectiveness of the pose over time.

THE POTENTIAL BENEFITS OF CONSISTENT SOMATIC EXERCISE PRACTICE

Consistent somatic exercise practice offers numerous potential benefits that can positively impact both the body and mind. Here are key advantages:

Physical Benefits:

• Improved Flexibility: Somatic exercises focus on mindful movement, gradually increasing flexibility by releasing muscle tension and enhancing joint mobility.

• Enhanced Body Awareness: Regular practice fosters a deeper connection between the mind and body, allowing individuals to better understand and sense bodily movements, postures, and sensations.

• Better Posture and Alignment: Somatic exercises emphasize proper alignment, aiding in correcting imbalances and promoting a more aligned posture, reducing strain on muscles and joints.

• Reduced Muscle Tension: Mindful movement and relaxation techniques in somatic exercises help release muscle tension, easing stiffness and promoting relaxation.

• Increased Mobility and Range of Motion: By targeting specific muscle groups, somatic exercises can improve overall mobility and expand the range of motion in joints.

Mental and Emotional Benefits:

• Stress Reduction: Somatic exercises incorporate mindfulness and relaxation techniques, reducing stress levels by calming the nervous system and promoting a sense of relaxation.

• Enhanced Mindfulness: Regular practice cultivates mindfulness, allowing individuals to be more present in the moment and develop a greater awareness of their thoughts, feelings, and bodily sensations.

• Improved Body-Mind Connection: Somatic exercises facilitate a stronger connection between mental and physical states, fostering a deeper understanding of how emotions and stress manifest in the body.

• Promotion of Relaxation Response: Consistent somatic practice triggers the relaxation response, which can counteract the body's stress response, leading to overall relaxation and well-being.

• Better Stress Management: Through regular practice, individuals can learn effective techniques to manage stress, improving resilience and coping mechanisms.

Overall Well-being:

• Enhanced Sleep Quality: Somatic exercises, especially relaxation-focused practices, can contribute to better sleep quality by promoting relaxation and reducing tension.

• Mind-Body Harmony: By integrating movement, breath, and mindfulness, somatic exercises promote a sense of balance and harmony between the body and mind.

• Increased Energy and Vitality: Regular somatic practice can boost energy levels, reduce fatigue, and promote a sense of vitality by improving circulation and reducing muscular fatigue.

• Emotional Regulation: Developing greater body awareness can aid in emotional regulation, allowing individuals to manage their emotions more effectively.

• Long-term Wellness: Consistent practice contributes to long-term physical and mental wellness, providing tools for self-care and overall health maintenance.

Consistency is key to reaping the benefits of somatic exercises. Engaging in regular practice, even for short durations, can yield significant improvements in both physical and mental well-being over time.

PRECAUTIONS OR CONTRAINDICATIONS FOR SPECIFIC HEALTH CONDITIONS OR INJURIES

Somatic exercises, while beneficial for many, might not be suitable for individuals with certain health conditions or injuries. Here are precautions and contraindications for specific situations:

Precautions and Contraindications:

• Recent Injuries or Surgeries: Individuals with recent surgeries or acute injuries should avoid somatic exercises without proper guidance or clearance from a healthcare professional.

• Chronic Pain Conditions: Those with chronic pain conditions like fibromyalgia, arthritis, or chronic back pain should approach somatic exercises cautiously and seek guidance from a healthcare provider.

• Osteoporosis or Bone Health Issues: Certain somatic exercises involving deep twists or extreme stretches might not be suitable for individuals with osteoporosis or compromised bone health. Modifications are crucial.

• Pregnancy: Pregnant individuals should exercise caution and avoid intense or high-impact somatic exercises, especially those lying on the back for an extended period.

• Cardiovascular Issues: People with heart conditions, high blood pressure, or other cardiovascular problems should avoid intense or strenuous somatic exercises that might elevate heart rate or blood pressure without medical guidance.

• Neurological Conditions: Individuals with neurological conditions, such as multiple sclerosis (MS) or Parkinson's disease, should proceed cautiously and consult healthcare providers before starting somatic exercises.

• Severe Musculoskeletal Issues: Those with severe musculoskeletal issues, spinal cord injuries, or significant structural abnormalities should avoid movements that may exacerbate their conditions.

• Limited Mobility or Disabilities: People with limited mobility, disabilities, or chronic health issues should seek guidance from healthcare professionals or experienced instructors for adapted exercises.

• Professional Guidance: Always consult a healthcare provider or certified somatic exercise instructor before starting a new exercise program, especially if you have underlying health concerns.

• Listen to Your Body: Pay attention to your body's signals. If a movement causes pain, discomfort, or feels unsafe, stop immediately and seek guidance.

• Start Slowly: Begin with gentle movements and progress gradually, especially if you're new to somatic exercises or recovering from an injury.

• Modify as Needed: Modify exercises to suit your individual needs or limitations. Use props, decrease intensity, or opt for alternative movements when necessary.

• Avoid Overexertion: Avoid pushing too hard or overexerting yourself, as this could lead to injury or exacerbate existing conditions.

• Stay Hydrated and Comfortable: Maintain hydration and wear comfortable clothing suitable for movement to ensure a pleasant exercise experience.

Individuals with specific health concerns or injuries should always consult healthcare professionals or qualified instructors before starting a new exercise regimen, including somatic exercises, to ensure safety and appropriateness for their individual circumstances.

HOW TO MOTIVATE YOURSELF TO CONTINUE PRACTICING AND EXPLORING SOMATIC EXERCISES

Staying motivated to continue practicing and exploring somatic exercises can be achieved through various strategies. Here are some effective ways to maintain motivation:

• Set Clear Goals: Define specific and achievable goals for your somatic practice. Whether it's improving flexibility, reducing stress, or enhancing body awareness, having clear objectives helps stay focused.

• Start Small and Consistent: Begin with manageable sessions. Even short daily practices can yield significant benefits. Consistency is key; commit to regular practice to experience gradual improvements.

• Explore Variety: Keep your practice interesting by exploring different somatic exercises, movements, or variations. Trying new techniques can prevent monotony and keep you engaged.

• Mindful Approach: Embrace mindfulness during practice. Be present in the moment, focus on sensations in your body, and observe the effects of each movement. This can deepen your connection with the exercises.

• Track Progress: Maintain a journal to track your progress, noting any improvements, insights, or challenges. Reviewing your journey can be motivating and encouraging.

• Find Inspiration: Seek inspiration from somatic practitioners, instructors, or online resources. Watching demonstrations, reading about the benefits, or engaging with a supportive community can boost motivation.

• Create a Dedicated Space: Designate a comfortable and calming space for your practice. Having a dedicated area can make it easier to commit to regular sessions.

• Practice Gratitude: Cultivate gratitude for your body's abilities and the opportunity to practice somatic exercises. A positive mindset can enhance motivation and enjoyment.

• Enjoy the Process: Focus on the experience and how your body feels during and after practice rather than just the end results. Appreciate the journey of exploration and learning.

• Reward Yourself: Celebrate small milestones or achievements in your practice. Reward yourself with something enjoyable to reinforce your commitment.

• Listen to Your Body: Respect your body's signals. If you're fatigued or experiencing discomfort, it's okay to take breaks or modify exercises to suit your needs.

• Accountability and Support: Find a practice buddy or join a somatic exercise group. Sharing experiences, discussing challenges, and supporting each other can boost motivation.

• Reflect on Benefits: Remind yourself of the benefits you've experienced through somatic practice. Whether it's reduced stress, increased flexibility, or better body awareness, reflect on how it positively impacts your life.

By integrating these strategies into your routine, you can maintain motivation, sustain your somatic practice, and continue exploring new aspects of mindful movement for overall well-being.

CONCLUSION

In conclusion, somatic exercises offer an accessible and transformative path for beginners embarking on a journey toward enhanced body awareness, improved flexibility, and holistic well-being. Rooted in the principles of mindful movement, these exercises facilitate a deeper connection between the mind and body, promoting relaxation, mobility, and a heightened sense of self-awareness.

For beginners, somatic exercises provide a gentle entry point into exploring movement with an emphasis on conscious awareness, breathing, and gradual progression. Through consistent practice, individuals can cultivate a more harmonious relationship between their physical and mental states, fostering relaxation, stress reduction, and improved posture.

The beauty of somatic exercises lies in their adaptability. Beginners can tailor their practice to suit their unique needs, gradually exploring various movements, gentle stretches, and mindfulness techniques to nurture their bodies. Starting slowly, listening to one's body, and embracing a mindful approach foster a supportive environment for growth and progression in somatic practice.

As beginners delve deeper into somatic exercises, they will discover the profound impact these practices can have on their overall well-being. The journey of exploration, learning, and self-discovery within somatic exercises is not solely about mastering postures but rather about fostering a deeper connection with oneself, leading to a more balanced and mindful way of living.

In embracing somatic exercises as a beginner, one not only embarks on a physical journey of movement and flexibility but also opens doors to emotional balance, stress reduction, and a heightened sense of mindfulness. The key lies in patience, consistency, and a willingness to embrace the process, allowing beginners to savor the transformative benefits that somatic exercises offer on the path to a more connected and harmonious life.